Stud AA7e NOS

AF899881

TELEPEN

11 0000416 9

3

Medical Library
University of Bristol

THIS BOOK/JOURNAL MUST BE RETURNED TO THE LIBRARY BY THE LAST DATE STAMPED BELOW.

THREE MONTHS
STACK
LOAN

UNIVERSITY OF BRISTOL

25 NOV 2019

WITHDRAWN

# Medical science and human goals

*For Lyn*

# Medical science and human goals

G. J. V. Nossal, CBE

Edward Arnold

© Brickell Nominees Pty. Ltd. 1975

First published 1975
by Edward Arnold (Publishers) Ltd.
25 Hill Street, London W1X 8LL

Boards edition ISBN: 0 7131 4247 2
Paper edition ISBN: 0 7131 4248 0

By the same author:
*Antibodies and Immunity* Penguin Books
*Antigens, Lymphoid Cells and the Immune Response* (with G.L. Ada).
Academic Press

All rights Reserved. No part of this publication may be reproduced, stored in a retrieval system, or transmitted in any form or by any means, electronic, mechanical, photocopying, recording or otherwise, without the prior permission of Edward Arnold (Publishers) Ltd.

UNIVERSITY
OF BRISTOL
MEDICINE

Photoset, printed and bound
in Great Britain by
REDWOOD BURN LIMITED
Trowbridge & Esher

# Preface

The nature and content of this book can best be foreshadowed by a consideration of the motives behind its writing. People in general are extremely interested in health (particularly their own!) and intensely curious, though in a rather general way, about progress in medical science. In the last half-century, medical science has at last justified this interest and has contributed in a powerful way to individual well-being and social development. Yet, the lines of communication between medical scientist and concerned layman remain poor; the knowledge that most people have of the scope of medical research is very sketchy. This is a bad thing, not only because a grasp of the nature of scientific research can be personally enriching, but also because modern science has become very expensive, and the layman who supports it financially has a right to accurate information. I believe a large part of the blame for this communication gap rests with the scientists. As a group, scientists have a large desire and need to communicate with each other, and this seems to erase the urge to communicate with outsiders.

One result of this general attitude is that much of the massive and frequently impressive literature on the history and philosophy of science has both a style and a content more suitable for insiders, for scientists and advanced students, than for a wider audience. Another consequence of practical importance is that medical and science students, when considering research as a possible career, find it difficult to gain information about the human aspects of such a calling. Their ideas of what it might be like, from day to day, are much less precise than their concept of a surgeon's life, or an engineer's.

It thus seemed to me that there was a place for a book about medical science written from the inside but for consumption largely on the outside. Moreover, I felt that an analysis of the role of medical science in social development and the future of man could only be illuminating if it dealt accurately with the qualities of mind and spirit, and with the aspirations and motivations of scientists. Thus the theme of scientists as people will recur frequently. Finally, I felt that several recent popular works on trends in medical research had painted an unnecessarily lurid picture of the future, at least the immediate future, and thus I have included some examples of actual or impending discoveries in my own field to illustrate both the accomplishments and the limitations of medical science.

Medical research today comprises a wide spectrum ranging from fundamental science to applied clinical research but embracing also newer fields forming a bridge to the social sciences. For example, medical sociology, psychology, operational research into systems of health care delivery and evaluative analysis are all assuming greater importance. My own life and experience has been more in laboratory and clinical sciences, and therefore treatment of these latter areas is necessarily cursory. This does *not* imply a denigration of their undoubted importance.

It is my hope that this book will appeal to a general lay audience and perhaps particularly to those laymen in decision-making positions in a democracy. It should be of interest to University students from the 'two cultures' and to school-leavers keen to think seriously about their lives and careers. If it falls into the hands of my colleagues in medical research, I hope they will conclude that I have painted our profession with accuracy, tolerance and some wit.

I am deeply indebted to Dr Margaret Pierce, Archivist to The Walter and Eliza Hall Institute of Medical Research, for considerable research assistance. I am also most grateful to Miss Lauretta Stokes, Mrs Vicki Adams and Miss Leonie Maxwell for their cheerful and painstaking typing of the manuscript.

G.J.V.N.

Melbourne, 1975

# Contents

# 1

# The nature of scientific discovery

*'The same thrill, the same awe and mystery, come again and again when we look at any problem deeply enough. With more knowledge comes deeper, more wonderful mystery, luring one on to penetrate deeper still. We turn over each new stone to find unimagined strangeness . . . it is true that few unscientific people have this particular type of religious experience'.* R. P. Feynman

## The knowledge continuum

The aim of science is a comprehension of the observable universe and all it contains, 'by the use of a minimum of primary concepts', as Einstein has put it. In other words, science attempts to explain the complex things that we perceive with our senses in terms of simpler elements that make up the perceived entity, and in terms of rules that govern the behaviour and relationships of the simpler component parts. Medical science seeks a comprehension of the human being in health and disease. It strives to know what makes the healthy human organism tick, to discover what portion of the system has failed in particular diseases and why, and to find ways of partially or completely repairing the fault. A scientific discovery consists of the demonstration of either a new component part or a new relationship between known component parts, and this can be achieved by experimental manipulation of the object of study, by theoretical deduction, or, most frequently, by a combination of the two.

The idea that will be most unfamiliar to the non-scientist is the open-ended nature of the situation. Despite the many hundreds of thousands of people around the world now engaged full-time in research, no one has yet fully solved a scientific problem. Further striving for logical connections between the object of study and the rest of nature is always possible. Let us illustrate this pessimistic-sounding notion with an example derived from medical research. Consider the problem of an attack of pneumonia. At first look, we might say that this problem is solved when we know that pneumonia is caused by the growth of certain bacteria in the lungs of the patient, and when we find and administer an antibiotic that kills the germ but does not harm the patient. But wait a moment: where did the pneumonia germ come from, and why did it attack that person and not his wife, who was with him almost constantly that week-end when he caught the pneumonia? Why does the germ attack the lungs and not the stomach or liver? Why does the antibiotic kill the germ but not the patient? In a twinkling, we realize that our first look did provide *a* solution, but by no means a *complete or final* one.

It is frequently stated that biological science today is in the same state that physics was in the early 1930's, not yet very advanced but on the threshold of a great leap forward. This superficial oversimplification irritates me considerably, not only because of its arbitrariness, but because it neglects this fundamental issue of open-endedness, of layers within layers of understanding. Physics leapt forward in the 'thirties because much was found out about the particles making up an atom and the energy relationships between them, but it was clear, then as now, that the increasing understanding gained was part of an ancient and continuing quest. Medical science seeks to understand a person in terms of the organs (brain, heart, kidney and so on) which make him up and the rules allowing those organs to function in harmonious unison. A great branch of medical science, namely physiology, deals with the function and interrelationship of the different organs, but of course each organ is made up of cells arrayed in highly specific patterns, and another science, histology, deals with this aspect. Cells in their turn are made up of definite parts called organelles, such as the nucleus and the powerhouses which we term mitochondria, and many more. These organelles in their turn are made up of molecules, many of which are very large. The large molecules, such as proteins or nucleic acids, are strings and coils of smaller molecular building blocks occurring in a defined number and sequence. Of course, these molecules act on each other in the cell; their interactions, physical and chemical, drive the life process along. The two sciences of biochemistry and biophysics consider the reactions taking place between biologically active molecules, and are usually regarded as the most fundamental level of biology. However, if the reader has followed my reasoning, he will soon see that this is quite an arbitrary end point. Obviously, molecules are made up of atoms, atoms of particles, and so we can work our way 'down' to chemistry, physics and mathematics. Equally obviously, people are parts of families, families of societies, societies of nations, nations of the world; and so we work our way 'up' from medicine to sociology and political science. While few, if any, scientists are professionally involved at all of the interfaces which exist in this hierarchy of disciplines, all encounter one or more in their work. I feel sure all would agree with my experience that the interface is at best a convenience; conventions dictate that certain phenomena, certain ways of describing or looking at things, are placed within one discipline. This facilitates teaching and erects the framework in which necessary specialization can develop, but it is important to realize that the different disciplines *are* conventions, and no more than that. In reality, the degree of continuity achieved in our knowledge is a measure of the success of science as a whole. In the portion of the continuum which we term medical science, the interdisciplinary bridge-building has been quite remarkable; the biologist need not feel ashamed in front of the physicist.

Therefore, the first great principle which we must consider is that knowledge and insight grow continuously as layers within layers of complexity are revealed by scientific discovery. The idea is not new, as over 300 years ago René Descartes wrote: 'All things to the knowledge of which man is competent are connected'. This was in fact written shortly before Newton's work paved the way for the rise of the experimental method. Since then, vast new continents of facts and laws have emerged through experimentation, which have changed the balance of power between man and his environment, and which as far as we can see are almost infinitely extensible. The further we go, the more we become impressed with the interconnectedness of things.

## The paradox of partial insight but total power

It should now be clear that the degree to which knowledge has advanced in any area of medicine is always relative, yet it does not follow that the power generated by the new knowledge need be only partial. Reverting to the simple example of our pneumonia case, the partial knowledge about the particular infective event is nevertheless sufficient for a complete cure. In other words, partial insight can be used for effective action. In most clinical situations, there remains an empiric element to treatment, which can be quite substantial; there comes a time when a sufficient number of the layers of complexity have been peeled off to allow an intelligent manipulation. In Chapter 9 we shall be considering several examples of major discoveries influencing the practice of medicine, but here my chief purpose is to explain that there is not a simple one to one relationship between depth of scientific understanding and ability to effect important social change. We have cases of relatively incomplete problem resolution with major usable consequence, and of course the opposite situation can also occur. It is important to stress this 'insight-power' paradox, because armed with this concept and with that of the 'knowledge continuum', much that would otherwise be obscure about the activities of scientists becomes clarified. Simply put, any aspect of biology can affect any other, and we cannot know in advance what breakthrough will emerge next.

## Levels of the nexus

What we have said so far implies that medical science is like an enormous three-dimensional jigsaw puzzle, with individual scientists working to fit pieces largely into a single layer but retaining the ability to jump up and down between the layers at least occasionally. We have concluded that the final structure will probably never be built, but that the players' quintessential ambition is to make the building into a compact, unlayered, continuous whole. We have also found that between the unfilled gaps of the puzzle we find islands of construction of great beauty and strength. Let us now examine the layers, unwelcome entities though they may be, in somewhat greater detail. This will necessitate a brief excursion into popular science and will introduce a few technical elements, but it is an essential prelude to the more interesting portion of this chapter which will seek to establish how and where new knowledge is born.

The most straightforward way to describe the professional activities of scientists working in the various layers is to take them in the sequence in which medical students learn subjects in the traditional British system. The inclusion of physics and chemistry stresses that biological systems consist of matter, but the treatment of these two subjects is necessarily superficial in a medical curriculum and even the widest definition of medical research usually excludes most projects in physics and chemistry. However, one branch of chemistry does qualify, and that is organic chemistry, or the chemistry of molecules derived from animals or plants; similarly, one branch of physics, termed biophysics, exists which applies the methodology and conceptual framework of physics to biological problems. Biophysics may encompass fields as diverse as the use of very fast spinning-machines (centrifuges) to separate protein molecules from each other; the analysis of the pumping action of the heart and the elasticity of blood vessels to discover what factors go to make up blood pressure; or the properties of X-rays, which allows them to penetrate cells. These two sciences of organic chemistry and biophysics are usually regarded as the bridges between the two great branches of the natural sciences, namely the physical and the biological.

At an equally early stage, medical students are introduced to cell biology. From a study either of very lowly life forms consisting of just one cell, or from an observation of cells taken from higher organisms but placed into simple, artificial growth conditions in plastic or glass dishes, they learn the role of the different parts of a cell. The traditional tool of cell biology is the microscope, now increasingly aided by the electron microscope, which can magnify cells up to half a million times. Once a cell was believed to consist only of a nucleus and of cytoplasm, but now we can recognize hundreds of different types of structures within cells, arranged in myriads of different patterns in cells with various functions. From cell biology, we move on to botany and zoology which deal with the way nature has built from this basic building block of a cell, the more complex forms of the plant and animal kingdoms. Genetics, the study of how properties of organisms are handed down to the progeny, is also taught at this early stage.

In his second and third years, the student moves on to anatomy, biochemistry and physiology. Traditional anatomy consists of dissecting the human body and learning where the different organs live, but in modern curricula the framework is much wider and more interesting than that. For example, microscopic anatomy or histology deals with the patterned organization of different cells in the various organs and tissues, and neuroanatomy relates the parts of the brain to specific functions such as thought, vision, speech or movement. Embryology seeks to determine the way a single cell, the fertilized egg, gradually develops into a whole human being. Whereas anatomy deals with the structure and location of organs, the closely related science of physiology deals with their function. It asks *how* the stomach absorbs food, *how* the nerves transmit signals from the brain to the muscles, *how* the kidneys purify the blood stream. Biochemistry deals with the chemical reactions going on inside cells and with the nature of the great biological polymer molecules such as nucleic acids, proteins, carbohydrates and fats. It must be obvious on even the most casual examination that these three great branches of learning overlap most extensively.

Traditionally, the above subjects constitute the 'pre-clinical' medical subjects, as they deal exclusively with normality. They are taught alike to medical, dental, veterinary science and science students, though in various ways and with differing emphases. Three practical consequences flow from this separation of 'pre-clinical' from the 'clinical' subjects studied in the later years. First, many governmental granting agencies supporting science classify research done in the pre-clinical subjects as 'scientific' and that done in clinical subjects as 'medical', as if the two were mutually exclusive. Secondly, a career involvement in the pre-clinical sciences frequently involves obtaining a Ph.D. degree, as opposed to the clinical 'M.D.' or 'M.B., B.S.'. Thirdly, many young medical students, thirsting for a direct involvement with sick people regard the pre-clinical sciences as a dry preliminary to the 'real' work which begins when they see patients. It is reassuring to note that in all three cases the barriers are beginning to break down. Granting agencies are increasingly recognizing the difficulty of distinction, the 'M.D. – Ph.D.' functions are becoming increasingly overlapping, and many medical schools are integrating curricula so that students see patients earlier and continue for longer their study of normal biological phenomena.

There are five major subjects taught in the clinical years and they are pathology, microbiology, pharmacology, medicine and surgery. Pathology deals with the way in which human organs change in structure, function and microscopic appearance when struck with any of the thousands of known separate diseases. Microbiology deals with man's parasites, viruses, bacteria, molds and tiny animals which infect or infest, and with the damage that this causes. My own science of immunology, which studies the body's ways of defending itself, is usually regarded as a branch of microbiology, though it undoubtedly contains large elements of physiology and pathology as well. Pharmacology is a study of chemical compounds called drugs which influence either a physiological function or a disease process. Medicine deals with the classification and recognition of human diseases in living patients, and with non-surgical treatment. Surgery deals with mechanical ways of repairing injuries or correcting defects or diseases. It goes without saying that many branches of both medicine (such as psychiatry, paediatrics or dermatology) or surgery (such as obstetrics or ophthalmology) are sufficiently distinctive as to require teaching in separate courses.

## The nature and scope of medical research

We are now in a position to define medical research, because it is simply all scholarly activity which deals with any of the areas of study outlined above, most definitely including, in my view, all of the biosciences pertaining to the pre-clinical curriculum. Any work leading to a deeper understanding of biological processes and hence of man as a biological entity sooner or later, directly or indirectly, impinges on some aspect of modern medical treatment.

I am frequently and deeply amazed, and indeed perturbed, at how little even educated people realize this wide scope of medical research. The thought that someone is seeking a cancer cure or a blood pressure-reducing pill comes readily into clear focus. However, the realization that someone like myself, as director of a medical research institute, should spend the major part of his life trying to work out how white blood cells of perfectly healthy mice manufacture antibodies arouses responses varying from disbelief through faint disappointment down to boredom or even pity! Admittedly this response pattern is changing as efforts to create greater community awareness of science increase, but there is still a very great contrast between the instant recognition of the importance of continued basic research by any medically or scientifically-trained person, and the rather laboured acceptance of the connection by the layman. As we shall consider fully in Chapter 8, this leads to grave errors of attitude and behaviour on both sides at the very time when clear communication is important.

There is, of course, a very large and important segment of medical research which does correspond to the popular image. This is called clinical research. Here, patients with a particular disease are the direct and immediate objects of study. Through a variety of specialized tests, which will include X-rays, blood examinations of complex and multi-facetted nature, microscopic viewing of little bits or 'biopsies' of diseased tissue, and many other elaborate explorations, the investigator seeks to come to as deep an understanding as possible of the cause of a disease, and of its relationship to other known diseases. Moreover, through prolonged study of a large number of cases of the same disease, the clinical researcher learns the likely outcome or 'prognosis' and can assess the efficacy of new treatments. It is a curious thing that in many University circles, clinical research is regarded as intellectually not very challenging. In fact, I regard it as the hardest form of medical research. The investigator must at all times have as his prime consideration the well-being of the patient. This naturally and properly limits severely the range of things he can do by way of investigation. Moreover, unlike the basic scientist who can breed up or purchase 1,000 mice without great difficulty, the clinical investigator cannot order large numbers of patients with his pet disease to appear suddenly at the door of his clinic, and indeed, case numbers are often the limiting factor in some aspects of his work. Finally, while the basic scientist can, if he wishes, choose to ignore possible applications or relevance of his work to disease problems, sure in the knowledge that someone else will apply his discovery when the time is ripe, the clinical researcher must always keep a watching brief on the advances made in the basic laboratory, because it will be from there that most of his cues will come. Thus, in general terms, clinical research tends to move more slowly than fundamental biology. This is one reason why many clinical investigators do a certain amount of laboratory work on experimental animals as well.

The medical scientist who works purely in a laboratory setting has fewer constraints on his activities and thus can range as widely or as deeply in his study of the phenomenon of current interest as his imagination and available resources will allow. This is probably the reason why the very best brains in science tend to be drawn into the basic fields, and a partial explanation of why the vast majority of Nobel Prizes in medicine have gone to workers who never go near real patients. The new principles of biology which create whole movements of consequent research and discovery almost always come from studies done on laboratory animals or smaller life forms. In effect, many medical scientists maintain a great interest in the interface between basic laboratory and hospital clinic.

There is one aspect of this interface important to an understanding of medical research. It is the concept of models of human disease in experimental animals. The most important goal of medical research is the prevention and treatment of human diseases. Obviously, most new drugs or treatments conceived in the mind of an investigator carry one or both of two risks. First, the new treatment may be ineffective or less effective than other known treatments. Secondly, it may carry some risk of an unwanted or even unsuspected injurious side-effect. Models of human diseases created artificially in experimental animals are vital tools in the chain of processes needed for the discovery and testing of new treatments. There are two types of model diseases to consider. The first is the spontaneous emergence of a disease which resembles a human disease. For example, I have in my laboratory mice which have been specifically inbred so as to yield a high incidence of leukaemia, or of anaemia, or of a specific type of kidney disease. The second type is where the investigator does something to an initially healthy animal to make it sick. For example, he might put a clip on to the artery supplying blood to the kidney of a rat, and the consequent reduction in blood flow will cause kidney disease and high blood pressure. Both sorts of models are extensively used in drug testing. Of course, the model is never an exact counterpart of the human malady, and no matter how carefully tests of both efficacy and toxicity of a new drug have been carried out in the experimental animal, the first application to man is still hazardous. A slow and arduous progression of clinical trials must take place before the real value of the new drug can emerge.

## The starting point for discovery

A discovery never comes out of the blue. Let me illustrate this by an example from the life of the man who was probably the most original thinker of the last half-millenium and the most important individual in the development of science, Isaac Newton. Princeton historian C. C. Gillispie proclaims that 'the mind of Sir Isaac Newton was one of the glories of the human race, and one of its mysteries'. In a scant eighteen months in 1665 and 1666, while the plague was raging in Cambridge, he discovered the law of gravity, the composition of light and the calculus, thus sketching the outlines that would contain physics for over 200 years. However, legends of falling apples notwithstanding, Newton had much to build on. Newton learnt from the planetary laws of Galileo (who died in 1642, the year of Newton's birth), the optics of Kepler, the cosmic picture of Descartes. He wrote somewhat grudgingly of his debt to the Dutch scientist Christian Huygens in the field of centrifugal force, and though he quarrelled greatly with Robert Hooke, the latter's fine experimental observations on light must have influenced Newton's thinking. Galileo, in his turn, did not arise in a scientific vacuum, but out of a substantial, traceable tradition. The British Historian Herbert Butterfield has shown clearly how much Galileo owed to figures such as Jean Buridan, Nicholas of Oresme and Albert of Saxony. These thinkers based their work on the ancient principles of Aristotle, Archimedes and Euclid. In fact, Butterfield makes out a persuasive case, qualifying the traditional concept of the Renaissance, for a continuous development of western thought from the eleventh or twelfth century. As far back as we can trace the history of discovery, the pattern has been to build on the achievements and insights of the past. This is not to say that the progression is linear, or to deny the reality of great quantum jumps, but if we would honestly seek the starting point for a discovery, it must needs be in a prior discovery.

Thus traditions are vastly important in research, and pervade its structure. Translating this to a contemporary setting, if a medical scientist wishes to discover something, to do research into a particular field or disease, he must first read, at least in part, the relevant scientific literature. This can and need rarely be complete, and must never be uncritical. Many of the finest discoveries have as their starting point the entry of a bright, relatively unschooled investigator, lacking firm preconceptions, into a new field. He brings to the problem not only this fresh approach but also a new research methodology or at least ideas for the construction of a new methodology. Good ideas (new and speculative syntheses concerning a problem) and good research methods are equally important to a worthwhile discovery.

Much insight into how research scientists work can be gained by considering the way that they report their findings to their colleagues. These days, oral communication through symposia, conferences and congresses is very important, but all scientists agree that the definitive description of a discovery must be in the form of a written report published in the open literature. The report which describes for the first time in definitive form a series of experiments and deductions leading to some conclusions is called a paper. The anatomy of a scientific paper is revealing. It begins with an introduction, in which the writer briefly lays out the subject to which he is addressing himself and annotates previous work done in the field. Next comes a section called 'Materials and Methods', in which the scientist sets out the tools of research which he has used in sufficient detail for any competent worker to come along and repeat the experiments described. In the next section of 'Results', we find an objective report of the results obtained in the experiments, usually including information on how frequently each experiment was repeated and how much variation was encountered from experiment to experiment. This section is (or should be) free of inferential or deductive material – it is the place where the reader finds the bald facts of the work done. In the last major section, the 'Discussion', the author is encouraged to let his hair down. Here he interprets the results in the light of what he or others have done previously in the field; he attempts to resolve any discrepancies; he draws conclusions, makes predictions and generalizations, and in short attempts to show how his little piece fits into the large jigsaw puzzle. The discussion can be the most interesting part of the paper. All the sections are liberally annotated with references to other people's work, and every paper ends with a list of detailed literature citations which enable the reader to check on any related aspect which may interest him. The paper also usually has a brief summary which capsulizes the highlights. Groups of papers make up a scientific journal, and issues of journals appear at intervals varying from weekly to quarterly. This whole elaborate and highly stylized process of publication of results is crucial to the development of science and as we shall see in Chapters 4 and 5, to the careers of individuals.

A short aside on other types of research publications may be helpful here. The lay reader will be familiar with textbooks, but may find it hard to realize that the standard University textbook really enters very little into the working life of scientists. Textbooks are syntheses of whole, large areas of knowledge. They are thus useful ways of gaining access to a new major subject about which one knows little, but they are usually not sufficiently detailed or up-to-date to help a scientist plan his next experiment in his own field. On the other hand, original papers of the sort I have described above are always highly specialized, and appear in frighteningly large numbers. Therefore there exist so-called 'reviews', an important type of publication where a reviewer draws together the chief results and conclusions of some scores to hundreds of papers dealing with a group of related problems. In my own field of immunology and transplantation biology, some scores of major important reviews appear each year! These help significantly in allowing one to keep up-to-date in one's field. A variant on the single-author review is the publication in book form of a scientific conference, where a group of scientists has been drawn together, frequently from all over the world, to present papers on connected topics, and where discussion and criticism by the participants makes always amusing and sometimes valuable reading. The final bridge to the textbook is the so-called monograph, a book longer than the usual review of 20 to 100 printed pages, but too detailed and specialized to be of much interest to under-graduates. To complete the picture, there are journals devoted to very short papers, preliminary communications and abstracts; other journals which do nothing but print titles of recently-published papers; and elaborate computer-based cross-indexing and cross-referencing systems to help scientists find information on the results of their colleagues anywhere in the world.

## General features of research

Dr. Alan Gregg, former Director for the Medical Sciences at the Rockefeller Foundation, has defined research as a procedure or sequence of activities consisting of 'selecting, observing, recording, comparing, analyzing, classifying the phenomena, and finally deriving appropriate inferences and perhaps integrations'. He goes on to suggest that the hallmarks of a good research scientist include knowing what is worth observing, formulating a specific and precise problem with imagination, intuitive insight and ingenuity, and performing experiments dictated by clear and consecutive thought. There thus seem to be two clear portions to most research activities – reflection on a problem; and action designed to cross-examine nature, concentrating attention on the regularities that underlie the complexities of phenomena. In physics, the reflective side is sometimes the sole activity required of the scientist, and so we have a theoretical physicist. Such a man can make a monumental contribution, but eventually he depends on an experimentalist to confirm or deny his theory. In biology, it is much more usual for each research worker to be both theoretician and experimentalist, though different investigators have differing skills in the two directions. It is a further feature of most research fields that, as time goes on and knowledge grows more precise, less and less can be done by the use of the unaided senses, and more dependency on complex instrumentation and intricate experimental design develops. This in turn means a greater commitment of time to sheer learning of methodology, and so the professional increasingly crowds out the gifted amateur.

## Analysis of some real discoveries

We are now in a position where the nature of scientific discovery can best be illustrated by concrete and contemporary examples, and I have chosen some from the broad field of immunology. Three of the most widely-hailed scientific triumphs of the 1960's were the discovery of the structure of the antibody molecule; that of the function of the thymus; and the ability to perform kidney transplants successfully. Of necessity, the textbooks of the future will give major credit for each discovery to only very few people: Drs. G. M. Edelman and R. R. Porter for the first; Drs. J. F. A. P. Miller and R. A. Good for the second; and a slightly larger and more amorphous group for the third, prominently including names such as Sir Peter Medawar, and Drs. D. Hume, J. Merrill, J. Murray and J. Hamburger. The discoveries of these men were signal landmarks in my field. Let us see how each of them came about.

In 1798, the English general practitioner Edward Jenner empirically discovered that placing material from cowpox sores on to scratches in the skin of people produced mild, harmless sores and effectively prevented the volunteers from catching the dreaded and frequently fatal smallpox. Over half a century later, Louis Pasteur discovered that microbes were the cause of putrefaction and soon he developed the notion of the microbial origin of infectious diseases. He and his disciples developed vaccination procedures based on the injection of killed bacteria or detoxified bacterial products, thus not only providing a scientific base for Jenner's discovery but immeasurably extending its impact. It was not until 1892, however, that two scientists, Roux at the Pasteur Institute in Paris and von Behring in Germany, independently discovered that the state of immunity depended on the presence in the blood of molecules that were soon called *Antikörper* or antibodies. In the first half of the 20th century, these molecules became favourite toys for a succession of brilliant chemists, most notably Paul Ehrlich and Karl Landsteiner, who found out a great deal about their specific properties of combining with all sorts of materials foreign to the body. Yet little was found out about the chemical structure of antibody, because blood contained so many different kinds of proteins which were hard to separate from antibodies. A big step forward came from Scandinavia in the 1930's, with the development of instruments which could separate proteins on the basis of their molecular size and their net electric charge. Another very great help was the finding that certain rare cancers in man pour out into the bloodstream vast quantities of antibodies in very pure and homogeneous form. Serum from the cancer victim became a precious research tool. Still progress on structural analysis was slow, until it gradually dawned on Porter, Edelman and other workers that the antibody molecule was complex and had to be split up into smaller component parts before it could be analyzed. Using quite different approaches, the two scientists delicately split the large, unwieldy molecule into more manageable fragments, and over some years the true and very intricate pattern of composition was revealed. It is now known that each single antibody molecule consists of 4 to 20 interlinked sub-molecules or 'chains', as these are called. The chains are made separately in the cell but are hooked together before secretion. Moreover, each chain itself consists of from 2 to 5 continuous but distinct portions, only the end one of which is involved in the capacity of the antibody to neutralize a particular micro-organism or poison. Finally, each portion of each chain consists of 110 basic building blocks, known as amino-acids, arranged in a strictly scheduled sequence. In 1965, the German scientist Dr. N. Hilschmann was the first to present a complete sequence analysis of one of the smaller, 2-component chains of an antibody using a methodology developed by Sanger, Edman and others for different proteins, and in 1969 Edelman and his students presented the complete structural analysis of a whole antibody molecule. The unbroken, fluctuating skein of discovery went back 100 years, and I have in fact told only a small fraction of the story.

The saga of the thymus is somewhat different as it contains a larger element of chance. With the possible exception of the tiny pineal gland, the thymus was the last organ of the body to have its function discovered. It is quite a large organ, especially in children and adolescents, situated in the front of the chest behind the breastbone. For about 100 years it has been known that it consists largely of a type of white blood cell known as a lymphocyte – very similar in size and shape to the lymphocytes in the blood and the spleen known to be important in immune defences. Yet, strangely, the thymus did not form antibodies, and in adult mice and rats it could be removed surgically without apparent harm to the mice. One fascinating thing, however, was known of the thymus. Certain strains of mice show an appallingly high incidence of lymphatic leukaemia – 95% or more dying from this form of white blood cell cancer. If the thymus is removed surgically in such mice in early adult life, the leukaemia which would otherwise inevitably have developed is prevented. This phenomenon, which had been extensively studied by Dr. Jacob Furth and others years before, engaged Dr. Miller in the late 1950's. In his studies of leukaemia, he had occasion to remove the thymus from progressively younger mice, and finally one day he developed a technique for performing the incredibly delicate surgery on newborn mice, weighing one-thirtieth of an ounce and about half an inch long! When such mice grew up, they did not develop leukaemia, and indeed the whole original purpose of the experiment was soon put aside. What happened was that such animals initially grew healthily, but soon after weaning they stopped growing, became extremely sick, developed extensive infections and died. What a contrast to the operation as performed in adult life, which had proved quite harmless and in some circumstances, life-saving! Analyzing the situation, Miller soon realized that he had come, by serendipity, on to the real function of the thymus. Far from being an organ of antibody production, the thymus is a school where young lymphocytes are trained in their task of becoming immune defenders. When they have learnt their job, they are exported from the thymus into the bloodstream, ready for their seek-and-destroy mission. All of this happens in very early life, at which time the thymus is a crucial master-mind organ in the development of the immune apparatus. Thus Miller, a cancer research worker, revolutionized immunology overnight in 1961 when his studies were published, and of course he has remained an immunologist ever since. As is so often the case in modern science, other workers were on the scent, approaching the problem from quite different points of view, and particularly the group of Dr. R. A. Good made distinguished, independent contributions to a field which is still full of fascination today.

If the antibody story highlights traditions in science and the thymus work the interacting roles of chance and a prepared mind, then the massive research which has led to kidney transplantation illustrates each of these two forces in generous measure. In fact, three lines of work, initially quite independent, came together in the 1950's to create the new discipline of transplantation biology which flowered so much in the 1960's and has entered the 1970's full of hope and promise. One line began in England in the second world war, when plastic surgeon Thomas Gibson and zoologist Peter Medawar tried to do something about the treatment of burns. Skin grafted on to the burnt area from a volunteer or a cadaver provided a useful first-aid dressing, but within two weeks or so shrivelled up, died and fell off – Why? Medawar carried on his studies in rabbits and mice, and soon discovered that the graft failure was due to an attack by the patient's white blood cells (lymphocytes). In fact, the response to the transplant was an immunological one. The lymphocytes recognized the foreignness of the grafted skin and went about their job of destroying what they took to be an invasion from the outside world. Medawar saw clearly that for skin grafts to work, the immunological barrier would have to be beaten. The second complex skein came from the world of cancer research. In order to study how cancer cells grow, scientists wanted to have a method of serially transplanting tumours that emerged in animals such as mice. This would enable quantitative study of the cancer cells long after the initial mouse had died. It gradually became evident that this was possible when the tumour cells were transplanted to a mouse closely inbred to the one that had developed cancer. Grafts to other mice not genetically identical with the cancerous mouse simply did not grow. Two scientists, Dr. P. Gorer of London and Dr. G. Snell of Bar Harbor, Maine, and their schools patiently worked out the reason and discovered certain distinct genetic characteristics that determined compatibility between tissues – the so-called histocompatibility genes. It did not take long for this thinking to inter-link with the immunological work of Medawar. The third aspect of the drama involved medical courage and surgical expertise. At the Peter Bent Brigham Hospital in Boston, a famous centre for the treatment and study of kidney diseases had grown up, but many kidney disorders still proved fatal. A medical-surgical team, which included Hume, Merrill and Murray, faced with patients doomed to certain death, developed the operation of transplanting a new kidney to take over from the two diseased, destroyed ones. Imagine the feeling of triumph as the grafted kidney began to work and the patient retreated from death's door. How bitter must it have been to see, 10 days or so after grafting, the transplanted kidney begin to fail. The reader will have guessed the cause – much easier to grasp now than in 1955! Again the need was to beat the immune system. The three skeins had come together.

In 1975 as this book goes to press, and after a decade's research by at least 2000 qualified investigators, the problem is still not fully beaten, but the immunologist has learnt to use powerful drugs and treatments to keep the lymphocytes at bay; the geneticist has provided matching tests that help to match up donor and host as closely as possible; and the surgeon has devised quite fantastic procedures for grafting of virtually any vital organ. In the most favorable circumstances, kidney grafts succeed about 75% of the time.

I trust these three examples of real discoveries have revealed a little about the nature of scientific discovery; about the need for a blending of individual reason, deep learning, persistence, collegiality and good fortune that is required. It appears that this has always been so, but in our century the pace and extent of discovery have increased so much that we are in danger of forgetting the long history of western thought.

*Further reading*

Burnet, F. M. *Biology and the Appreciation of Life*. Sun Books, Melbourne (1968).
Butterfield, H. *The Origins of Modern Science 1300–1800*. G. Bell and Sons Ltd. London (1958).
Gillispie, C. C. *The Edge of Objectivity*: an essay in the history of scientific ideas. Princeton University Press (1960).
Oppenheimer, J. R. *Science and the Common Understanding*. B. B. C. Reith Lectures. Oxford University Press, London (1954).
de Solla Price, D. J. *Science since Babylon*. Yale University Press, New Haven (1961).
Wightman, W. P. D. *The Emergence of Scientific Medicine*. Oliver and Boyd, Edinburgh (1971).

# 2

# Specialization and generalization in science and medicine

*'Man can learn nothing unless he proceeds from the known to the unknown. . . . In biological sciences, the role of method is even more important than in the other sciences, because of the complexity of the phenomena and the countless sources of error'.* Claude Bernard

The fear is frequently expressed that ultra-specialization will lead to an eventual destruction of science. This view holds that there will be vast numbers of sub-disciplines, each with a tight-knit band of adherents. Individuals will know more and more about less and less; subspecialties will be separated from each other by insuperable language barriers; groups will tend increasingly to look inwards, and so forth. While there certainly are rational grounds to these fears, I personally take an optimistic stance on this issue. I believe an increasing number of unifying principles is emerging to further the competing cause of generalization in science. In this chapter, we shall examine the effects of both principles looking at both the light and the dark sides.

## Growth in scientific effort and specialization

In the last chapter, we stressed the continuity of science, both with respect to the roots of discoveries in prior discoveries, and from the viewpoint of inter-relatedness of disciplines. However, even the most cursory look through a science library will show that the amount of new scientific knowledge generated in the last few decades far outstrips the amount for the whole of previous history. It is, of course, not easy to measure discovery with accuracy. Howevei, a substantial research field has grown up which deals with 'the science of science', and which seeks in effect to put some numbers on this growth of science, which we all know intuitively to have taken place. One of the foremost experts in this area is Dr. Derek J. de Solla Price of Yale University, and his book 'Little Science, Big Science' explains much of what has happened. Growth in science, says de Solla

Price, has been progressing steadily for at least 200 years and probably longer, but the rate of growth has been exponential rather than arithmetic. What this means is that principles of compound rather than simple interest apply. It appears that by practically every criterion, such as number of people employed in research, number of new scientific journals, and amount of money spent on science, we have been for a considerable time on an upward climb of about 7% per annum, which means a doubling every ten years. If this is a correct figure, then the rate of effort in science in 1970 would have been 128 times greater than at the turn of the century. It is clear that such a growth rate cannot be maintained indefinitely, or else soon every person in the world would have to be a scientist! There have in fact been signs over the past 5 years of slowing in science expenditure, at least in the developed nations. However, it is clear that the universal acceptance of the methods of science as valid and efficient means of arriving at satisfactory solutions of problems is a phenomenon of the 20th century. A natural outgrowth of this has been a tendency for subject areas to bud off from the parent science of which they were originally a part. Once a science has assumed independent status, all kinds of pressures build up, both human and technical, for further internal growth and eventually for a repetition of the whole process. An understanding of this trend is very important, and thus a specific example may be helpful.

As in Chapter 1, let us draw our example from immunology. This clearly grew out of Pasteurian microbiology, but it was not long before the chemical side of the antibody problem became largely separated from the biological-medical side, and so the sub-science known as immunochemistry gained independent status. Today, immunochemistry itself is split into several camps. The same picture of extreme sub-specialization holds for organ transplantation, which field can be split into at least three parts: the surgical skills needed to perform technically perfect grafts; the medical part where physicians (rather than surgeons) try to shut off the immune rejection; and the field of organ preservation, where physiologists study how organs from cadavers might be preserved for future use. Next we can consider the cellular aspects of transplantation, where again operationally the researchers tend to split into two camps, reflecting two different kinds of lymphocytes involved in graft rejection. When we look at transplantation genetics, we see again that one sub-group is involved in the cell biology of this field, another in the biochemical aspects. So one could go on to classify and sub-classify, and could with no difficulty identify at least 20 sub-sciences within the broad umbrella of immunology, a field which has existed as such for a much shorter period than many sciences.

## The saving grace of unifying concepts

If this were the only side of the coin, the prophets of doom would probably soon be rejoicing. Let us look, then, at the other side; that of general concepts in biology and medicine. What is it, in essence, that separates the various sub-specialties described for immunology? It is chiefly an operational necessity during the rapid growth phase of scientific discovery for the use of highly specialized techniques and equipment, and for the development of a kind of informational shorthand, a special language or jargon, to accelerate communication between individual and geographically separated workers. In effect, as soon as a major piece of research has been fruitful, it is usually found that the concepts underlying the new finding are rather simple. The discovery can be explained effectively to non-specialists who would have had little interest in all the struggles that went into the discovery, or the many fruitless blind alleys encountered on the way. Therefore, at any one time, most scientists can have an operational, contributory interest in only a very few chosen sub-specialties; but can, with just a little extra effort, maintain a broad general interest. While this will by no means cover the whole gamut of the biological sciences, as might have been the case in the 19th century, it still ranges very widely. There are any number of vehicles using either the written or the spoken word, by which scientists can keep themselves broad, and the most effective weapon towards this desirable generalization of knowledge is a major unifying concept. When a really important discovery is made, it has such power, such appeal, such an aura of excitement around it, that it is very difficult to avoid becoming aware of it if one is professionally involved in science and even vaguely wide awake.

The best example of such a unifying concept in modern biology is the genetic code. In a little over a decade, the field of molecular biology totally and permanently altered the face of the biosciences. It was found that all the specifications for the sorts of molecules a cell, and thus an individual, could make were encoded in molecules of nucleic acid. One form of nucleic acid, called DNA, is the master copy of the instructions, and is the hereditary material passed on from cell to daughter cell, from generation to generation. The other form called RNA is an intermediary and discardable copy of portions of DNA. It moves from the nucleus of the cell to the cytoplasmic factories as a taped message of instructions. Then enzymes help to read the message and to construct the proteins, linking amino-acid after amino-acid according to a sequence exactly specified by the gene's DNA and in turn the messenger RNA. The basic outline of this scheme was the discovery of Drs J. D. Watson and F. H. Crick, and Dr Marshall Nirenberg and colleagues were able to 'crack' the code in exact form. Incredibly enough, there are only 4 basic symbols in the nucleic acid code. A sequence of three of these in a row will give $4 \times 4 \times 4$ or 64 code words, and this is more than enough to specify the 20 different amino acids. Some code words or 'codons' are used for start and stop signals, and in other cases two or more codons specify the same amino acid. The sequence of codons in the gene therefore determines the sequence of amino acids in the protein. Dr C. Anfinsen and others have established that the actual shape in three-dimensional terms of a protein molecule is totally determined by the amino-acid sequence. Given a particular sequence, the resulting chain must fold in a particular way. Through a technique known as X-ray crystallography, we now have accurate three-dimensional models of many proteins, with the position of every one of thousands of atoms known. This reveals exquisite design features of the individual protein molecule, equipping each molecule for the performance of its particular task in the life process. All of this three-dimensional complexity is contained in the simple, linear array of the 4-symbolic triplet code. As the proteins in their turn are responsible for the construction of the other characteristic polymers of life, it will be obvious that directly or indirectly any aspect of the function of the cell will be affected by the molecular code mechanism. Potentially at least, every biological phenomenon will have a molecular explanation.

We are a long way from this kind of precision in many important branches of biology. The nature of thought and behaviour, the differences between cells of different organs, the regulation of growth and many other problems are not yet understandable in the language of this particular layer. Immunology, on the other hand, has already received enormous dividends from the molecular genetic approach. In either event, the genetic code has given new heart to investigators. It has acted as a tremendous unifying force; the beauty and essential simplicity of this aspect of nature's design, once revealed, will continue its fertilizing effect indefinitely. Already we have seen both 'upward' and 'downward' spread from the layer that we term molecular biology. It is spreading 'upwards' into cell biology and physiology, and 'downwards' as biophysicists and physical chemists study the nucleic acids in greater depth, fascinated and challenged by the prospects of understanding life in atomic terms. If a generalization of this degree of force emerges even once in a generation, it is sufficient in my eyes to dispel the gravest fears about overspecialization. Specialization has short-range, operational advantages necessary to the day to day conduct of research, but generalization is still an effective counterbalancing power, ever more necessary to the progress of biology as a whole. Conscious effort by scientists can maintain a reasonable balance between the two.

## Interdisciplinary synthesis and information spread

Insights as shattering as the cracking of the genetic code are, unfortunately, not too frequent. How is fragmentation and overspecialization avoided in the day-to-day life of working scientists? This depends largely on individual initiative and decision. At any given time, a researcher trying to solve a problem will usually restrict himself to a small number of experimental techniques, and he may well stick to this panoply for months or even years. Obviously, proper conduct of his research means that he must keep abreast of developments in other laboratories using these techniques and approaches, and thus almost by definition every scientist must do some reading of the technical literature. Fortunately, the information exchange media, be they scientific journals or societies arranging scientific meetings and symposia, have been vigorous in their efforts to promote broader scholarship in science. In other words, the working scientist who reads journals in a library or attends scientific meetings has his nose rubbed, as it were, in review articles and broadly-based lectures which seek to further generalization in science.

Another way in which rigid specialization is prevented might be termed 'technique cross-fertilization'. To study natural phenomena, scientists are always producing new machines with new analytical powers. It is frequently the case that a machine designed for one particular purpose turns out unexpectedly useful for quite a different one. For example, radioactive atoms and molecules were created in complex and expensive reactors primarily because the nuclear physicist wanted to study nuclear physics. These self-same 'radio-isotopes' as they are called, and the electronic and photographic devices which record their activity, have become indispensable tools of the biologist. In fact, without isotopes the molecular biology revolution could never have happened, and the cell biologist as well as practically every other type of medical scientist would be severely handicapped. Naturally, the scientist anxious to apply a new technique to his problem will first have to learn about the original application of the method. In so doing, he will perforce cross disciplinary barriers and contribute to the cause of generalization in science.

Another pattern of activity modifying the progression to overspecialization is the budding off of bridging disciplines. It frequently happens that a new research finding leads to the development of a branch of a science which simply does not fit into the established framework of existing disciplines. We have already seen how a sub-discipline can be created, but in the present case what frequently happens is the emergence of a new science which seeks to merge the best and most relevant features of two or more pre-existing sciences into its fabric. An example is present-day research into the brain and nervous system. The classical tools for studying the function of the brain were two-fold. First, there was anatomy (including microscopic anatomy) which sought in a somewhat static and pictorial way to describe the complex components of the nervous system. Secondly, there was neurophysiology, which looked at the brain primarily in terms of electrical circuitry. Both of these approaches have made splendid progress, but without giving anything like an intellectually-satisfying global picture of nervous system functioning. Then came the molecular biology revolution, and a group of extremely gifted men thought the time had come to use the insights gained in much simpler cellular systems for a study of the brain. Thus a new science was born – neurobiology, a synthetic mix of molecular biology, cell biology and neurophysiology. It is too early to tell whether this conscious adoption of a different disciplinary framework will lead to a better knowledge of how the brain works, but the very attempt is a bulwark against destructive over-specialization in science. It is pleasing to note that examples of such conscious attempts at interdisciplinary synthesis, both at the level of actual experimentation, and of symposia and monographs, are increasing in number and quality.

## Historical evolution of research fields: Openings through complexity to simplicity

How does a major line of scientific investigation actually begin? There are essentially two ways. Sometimes a scientist, engaged in theoretical analysis of his own or someone else's experiments, achieves a totally new synthesis or insight, suggesting a whole series of experimental tests of some new hypothesis. More frequently, a routine experiment performed as part of a continuing line of research, gives an unusual, unexpected result which urgently demands confirmation and follow-up with the gradual realization that a new frontier is emerging. The fact that this second pathway is the more common illustrates a number of important points. It reveals that greatness in science is somewhat a will o' the wisp; it is today quite rare for someone to sit in an armchair and design experiments that will lead to a great discovery. Much more commonly, the mantle falls on the thorough professional with the prepared mind and the material resources to follow up with vigour and imagination some unusual result.

Secondly, it illustrates that scientists can only be effective in an atmosphere of academic freedom, to follow their star into research fields possibly quite distant from the original experimental aim. Thirdly, it shows that even major turning-points in science are rarely appreciated instantly, but more frequently seep into the general scientific consciousness over a period of one to two years, thus giving the originator of the turning point, and/or a small number of other people, a chance to make substantial headway in research and to gain great prestige before the field becomes a 'bandwagon'.

Nothing is more exciting in science than to be caught up at the beginning of one of these turning points. All of a sudden, your life is in a whirl, your head buzzing with innumerable experiments; the days seem to have far too few hours and you begrudge sleep; your previous line of experimental work seems incredibly dull and you resent the need to polish it off in some sort of a way. But let us beware! This first phase is nearly always transient. The new insight or the unexpected result has created an opening. A blinding ray of light, pristine in its simplicity, is beckoning. A whole group of scattered facts and observations fall together, begin to dance an orderly minuet in your mind. You see six months or a year's experimental work laid out before you – that should 'wrap it up', you say. The next phase, however, will help to sort the men from the boys! In most new lines of research, the concept that initially seemed so clear and simple next becomes complex. Experiments that should have been confirmatory work out in the right general direction, but not black and white. Qualifying results come up that seem to limit the universality of your idea. Eight experimental animals behave as they should, but the other two give a seemingly opposite result. There follows a period, frequently of some years, when the new field which the ray of light has created becomes in its turn complex and turbid. This is not a flaw in the initial discovery but a manifestation of the intricacy of natural phenomena, and of our inability to penetrate all the layers of knowledge at one stroke. The beacon is indeed there, but when we open the door to the room from which it is issuing, we find the inner recesses of the room dark. We must now turn the beacon painstakingly into every corner, and this takes time. If the original discovery really was worthwhile, it will soon draw into the new research field numbers of workers who gradually study the many variables and bring the field to its second and genuine state of simplicity. At that stage, one more island of beauty and strength has been added to our ever-growing three-dimensional crossword puzzle.

We must distinguish this essential simplicity of the new principle from the great variety of detailed situations to which it can be applied. Thus, after the exciting 'honeymoon' phase of a research field, there is still much routine work to be done, which could be of the greatest practical importance. Turning again to immunology, we see that the great insight in the post-Pasteurian era was the fact that microbes, and products derived from them, stimulate the recipient person to form antibodies which neutralize the microbes. To apply this discovery to more and more of the common micro-organisms causing human disease required research of a high order. Though no longer world-shattering in its fundamental scientific content, it certainly was so in its human importance. We shall take up the relationship between pure and applied research in some detail in Chapter 3.

We have chosen above an example of worthwhile research still left to be done after the fundamentals of a new field have been settled. Unfortunately, one could also think of many examples of trivial research following in the wake of major discovery. This involves programming in minor, insignificant variations and elaborations into experiments, the fundamental outcome of which is predictable. After the growth phase of a new discipline, and once the fundamental principle has been thoroughly established, there follows this plateau period of research when no real progress is being made. In such a phase, it might be best to terminate this line of research and free the energies of the workers involved for different projects. However, this is never a simple matter. The phase of intensive growth will have brought into the field many people now committed to a particular technique, with vocational skills geared towards research of a particular character. Not all of these people will be able; some will be limited in their outlook; others may be ageing or have run out of steam; in short, many will be essentially incapable of starting the adventure all over again. Thus the research area will putter on, rapidly losing glamour as the oncoming generation of scientists, taking the original great discovery for granted, forges past looking for new fields to conquer. It is then important to take note of the new reality in the design of teaching curricula and in research grant funding.

## Fashions and bandwagons in science

This brings us on to a consideration of two profound, important phenomena in science namely the rule of fashion and the growth of bandwagons. The former is age-old and tied up with the concept of leadership. The latter is new to the era of 'big science' and warrants close scrutiny. At any given time, not every branch of science, nor even every inherently important field, attracts equivalent prestige and support. For reasons that are too multifactorial for facile analysis, some subjects capture the imaginations of the most gifted workers, attract the brightest students and receive the biggest government grants. There is usually a valid background to such a fashion associated with a basic discovery and real potential for rapid progress. Another aspect may be the dominance of a field by a heroic figure or even group of figures whose personal brilliance is the powerful beckoning force. Fashions, while they last, have their uses. They certainly represent one way of skimming the cream off a research area in the quickest time. They have their dangers, also, amongst the most prominent of which is the possibility that so many talented people will be brought into one branch of learning that one or more allied branches languishes for lack of attention. In time, however, this equilibrates out as the allied field, if important, will come to enjoy its period of high fashion in due course. Fashions that are based on real parameters, such as new integrating hypotheses, powerful new technologies, or a clearly major breakthrough, are a positive force in science.

Bandwagons, however, are another matter. In this context, I consider a bandwagon to represent the exploitation of a fashion beyond reasonable limits of usefulness by people of sub-optimal ability or motivation. In the era of 'big science', there are large numbers of people who elect to do research, or perhaps feel obliged to do some research while primarily engaged in another occupation, but who have little gift for discovery. There are others, more talented but unscrupulous, erratic or over-ambitious. Amongst these groups one finds the bandwagon-hoppers. As soon as it is clear that a particular research field will be prominent, they scurry to find some little corner on which they can do research. All too frequently, they do a half-hearted, superficial job and hop on to the next oncoming bandwagon, leaving a mess to be cleared up by some future researcher. I have nothing against a researcher who identifies a new field as being promising, and follows the fashion with genuine intent to make a serious contribution. On the other hand, to join whatever field happens to be most prominent for some short-term personal gain or evanescent thrill is a policy which, in the long run, works to the disadvantage of science as a whole and the happiness of the individual thus driven. There is a grave responsibility on those with policy-making power in research to distinguish fashions from bandwagons, and to temper fiscal enthusiasm for some new or popular field with the wisdom that regards worthwhile research essentially as a very long-term affair.

Who or what determines whether a discovery is important? This is one of the most difficult questions in science to answer. The criterion which the layman will apply most readily is its usefulness, yet many of the greatest discoveries have been entirely useless in the direct sense, and many useful findings have lacked the hallmarks of originality and depth needed for real greatness. One quality which seems to be important is the ability of a discovery to illuminate more than just a very restricted field – the capacity to penetrate to other layers of knowledge. Even more important is some difficult to define, intrinsic quality of the discovery which gives authoritativeness. This comes from the way the research is done. It requires a meticulousness and rigour which is such that it becomes a matter of great ease for another research group to duplicate and thus confirm the findings. Discoveries of this solid nature need not be global in their impact; they may simply represent useful bricks giving stability to the growing edifice. In fact, the reputations of most prominent scientists are built on discoveries of this nature, as it is given to few to break totally new ground. The final court of appeal on the importance of a line of research is the peer group. Important research is neither more nor less than what the recognized scholars, competent in the field, collectively deem to be important. This sounds shockingly arbitrary, and indeed some tragic mistakes of failure of recognition have occurred in the history of science. Nevertheless, it is the closest that we can come to an operational definition of what is important, and, as we shall see, the esteem of the peer group is one of the most cherished goals of working scientists.

## Specialization and generalization in medical research

So far we have said little in this chapter of specific significance for medicine. Medical research other than clinical research obeys most of the rules that we have discussed above. However, the clinical researcher faces one extra problem. He will be specialized not only by virtue of the research techniques he has mastered and the fields into which he has chosen to read in greatest depth, but he will also be practising that specialty on patients. In fact, the nature of his appointment (as an ophthalmologist or endocrinologist or psychiatrist) will usually specify the limits within which he must keep his desires for generalization confined. In real life, this necessary specialization is not as confining as it might appear. First, most of the clinical sub-specialities now represent vast fields of learning in their own right, allowing plenty of room for the exercise of creativity. Secondly, the clinical specialist frequently finds himself as part of a team in the management of a patient, thereby of necessity learning of progress in specialties other than his own. Thirdly, the clinical researcher may sometimes have the satisfaction of actually drawing the basic scientist's attention to some fundamental truth which the latter may then exploit to the full. For example, he may find that a drug has an entirely unexpected beneficial effect, which may reshape thinking in the relevant area of physiology; or else he may see that a disease process is an experiment of nature, giving insight into causal relationships that can subsequently be confirmed by animal experimentation. Finally, the clinical researcher has the satisfaction of the human aspect of his calling, and this can be more liberating than even the most general of scientific findings.

## Will generalization triumph?

No one will deny that formidable barriers exist to the eventual triumph of generalization in science. The capacity of the human brain is one factor, the continuation in many centres of teaching in rigid, discipline-oriented compartments is another. It is certainly far-fetched to think of one human being as an expert in every major branch of biological science. But is this necessary? As long as the knowledge continuum is maintained through a nexus of people each straddling one or two layers; as long as the historic trend of major branches of science is towards greater simplicity; as long as the leaders of science recognize the increasing need for inter-disciplinary synthesis; there seems to me no cause for despair. Scientists will have to become much more ambitious in their thinking about knowledge retrieval and dissemination systems, much more attuned to automation and also to a greater personal expenditure of energy in the cause of generalization. They will need to learn a quaint ambivalent attitude to knowledge, maintaining scrupulous depth and involvement in their own specialty while cultivating general and cursory acquaintance with developments in allied fields. Perhaps the greatest hope of all lies in wider community education. As generations whose lives are being increasingly shaped by science and technology come to dominate in the world, so the need for awareness of science, its benefits and perils, its triumphs and limitations becomes acute. Let us heed this imperative and strive in every way possible to comprehend science in the broadest framework.

*Further reading*

E. Borek, *The Code of Life.* Columbia University Press (1965).
C. R. Harington, *Leadership in Scientific Research.* Oxford University Press, London (1958).
P. B. Medawar, *The Art of the Soluble. Creativity and Originality in Science.* Methuen, London (1967).

# 3

# The institutional framework of pure and applied research

'*Science always has its two aspects, its intellectual aspect as knowledge and its practical aspect as control. . . . Every science arrives at a stage during which it makes its main broad contributions to practical human affairs. Biology is clearly on the verge of such a phase*'. Julian Huxley, 1931

We have seen that human knowledge is a continuum, but that to understand and describe it, we must break it up into arbitrary segments or layers. So far, we have studied these with respect to different branches or disciplines of learning. There is another way of breaking up scientific endeavour, in which a particular discipline is dissected into layers of increasing practical usefulness or applicability to human problems or needs. This break-up is described variously as 'pure' versus 'applied' research, 'research' versus 'development', 'science' versus 'technology' and in the field of medicine as 'basic' versus 'clinical' research.

In the higher centres of learning, I must with reluctance admit that a very great deal of nonsense is talked about pure versus applied research. There has been a sort of unwritten tradition that considers contributions to pure research as more admirable, more worthwhile, or reflecting greater intellectual ability. This is true when one considers a Newton, a Darwin, or an Einstein, because the major scientific revolutions depend on very fundamental new insights. However, for every figure of this dimension there will be tens of thousands of highly capable professionals engaged in research. With respect to the contributions that such individuals make, it has always seemed to me that pure and applied fields abound equally with challenging intellectual problems, the solution of which requires real ability and gives real satisfaction. It is my impression that the somewhat snobbish attitude of many academics to applied research may be, in part, responsible for the problems which Universities are facing today. There is little doubt that the man in the street, who after all foots the bill for research, finds it much easier to identify with applied aspects of research, where he can see a definite dividend emerging at the end. He is not right either, and the truth is that humanity will be best served if pure and applied research move forward in close parallel formation.

In this chapter, we will look at the institutional framework of pure and applied research, again from the viewpoint predominantly of biology and medicine. Our analysis can only be fruitful, however, if we recall that the distinction is arbitrary. In effect, every element in this particular continuum can and does feed back on every other. The 'purest' of ivory towers may discover a new principle which leads to a disease cure; equally, industrial research may unveil some precious fundamental. For example, the space race, an example of applied research, has led to revolutions in astronomy, astrophysics and geology; just as nuclear physics, originally the purest of pure research, has irrevocably altered the human condition by producing the information necessary for atomic and hydrogen bombs. If this qualification is borne in mind, we will understand the nature of research in the various institutions much better.

## Historical background to research backing by institutions

Research as a professional activity, extensively funded and being a major or sole preoccupation of an institution, is a very recent human activity. In particular, medical research, to the extent that it existed at all before the 19th century, was an irregular by-product of the activities of practising physicians. It is extraordinary to reflect on the fact that over the millenia since the ancient Greeks, physicians as a group made no deliberate effort to set up a regular machinery for questioning and assessing the value of their treatment or for a concerted search for better remedies. Even as late as the year 1900, it was common for University professors to engage in research essentially in their spare time and to have that research financed either out of their own pockets or through the kind offices of some rich friend who believed in them. From that point of view, then, the Universities represented the traditional institutions responsible for research, although unquestionably the learned societies, such as the Royal Society in London, the Academie Française or the Société Royale de Médecine in Paris, had a profound influence. Edward Jenner, for example, was a general practitioner with no institutional base. Louis Pasteur worked initially for the wine industry. The large, famous and well-supported research institutes are a phenomenon of the last 100 years. For example, the Pasteur Institute in Paris was opened in 1888, the Lister Institute in London in 1891, the world-renowned Rockefeller Institute in New York not till 1901. Then before World War I great national grant-giving organizations supporting research both in their own institutes and in Universities were

UNIVERSITY OF BRISTOL MEDICINE

born, including the British Medical Research Council in 1913 and the Kaiser Wilhelm Gesellschaft in Germany, which became the Max Planck Gesellschaft. Over this period, also, great influence for the good of medical research was exerted by the big American private philanthropic organizations. Foundations such as Carnegie, Rockefeller, Commonwealth and Ford had funds to spend in the first 30 years of this century that were quite enormous by the standards of the day, and in general they wielded their catalytic power in education with great imagination, grace and perspicacity. Indeed, in the United States the effectiveness of private financing of medical research acted as a major spur to greater efforts by Government.

World War II brought about a fundamental change in attitudes to research. Clearly, science and technology had been of decisive influence in determining the outcome of the war, and it became more generally recognized that research would be an equally shaping force for peaceful progress. As regards medical research, there was a greatly expanded expenditure through governmental agencies. Without any question, the pace-setter was a United States agency called the National Institutes of Health (NIH). This agency had an intramural programme of research at a very large research institute near Washington, but more importantly from our present viewpoint, it administered an extramural research grant programme through which investigators at Universities and other Institutions could receive funds for their work. The NIH budget grew prodigiously between 1950 and 1965, at the latter time being well in excess of $US 1 billion. This fiscal largesse on the part of the U.S. Government had global implications. Not only did some of the funds go to foreign grantees, but also the success of American medical research under adequate funding created imbalances which gradually became apparent to other countries, whose governments then accelerated medical research expenditure, though usually on a less lavish scale. We will be examining the role of Government policy in medical research more fully in Chapter 6. Here, I wish only to record that at the time of writing, government financing represents the sheet-anchor of virtually all world medical research projects except those sponsored by the pharmaceutical industry. Most importantly, it has become generally recognized that effective research requires the expenditure of substantial sums of money and that a nation wishing to make a real contribution must employ public funds for the purpose.

At the present time, there are therefore essentially three kinds of institutions engaged in medical research: medical research institutes; Universities; and industrial firms, chiefly pharmaceutical manufacturers. The purpose of the present chapter is to outline the diverse characteristics of these three, and the advantages and disadvantages of each.

## Medical research institutes

Most of the 'developed' nations of the world have one or more institutes, disengaged from the mainstream of University teaching, the chief or sole function of which is to perform medical research. While there is wide individual variation from country to country in the organization of such institutions, we can generalize to the extent that institutes are either governmental or private; and either mission-oriented or not. Examples of governmental research institutes are the National Institutes of Health in U.S.A. or the National Institute for Medical Research, Mill Hill, London. These are governmental to the extent that all their funds come from Government but, fortunately they have in most countries retained a large measure of institutional autonomy and independence from political influence. A second type of governmental research institute with which I am much less familiar, and which I shall therefore not discuss at length, is that where the aim of the research is more directly linked to other governmental programmes. Amongst these would be biological warfare institutions, epidemiological or pathological research institutes administered by the armed forces, research establishments associated with governmental vaccine-producing facilities, and so forth.

The private medical research institutes constitute a small and somewhat elite band of institutions, usually administered by a lay board of directors, incorporated as private, non-profit institutions, and arising originally through a philanthropic urge. Examples would include the Rockefeller Institute in New York (recently converted to the Rockefeller University); the Wistar Institute in Philadelphia; the Lister Institute in London and the Walter and Eliza Hall Institute in Melbourne. At their original inception, these institutions relied solely on private funds (donations, bequests, etc.) but over the last thirty years, they, too, have become increasingly dependent on government grants. To my knowledge, the only major medical research institute in the world which still exists solely from its endowment is the Carnegie Institute of Washington, which has five campuses, the activities of which are supported by the interest from the huge Carnegie legacy. Some important institutes are difficult to classify, being largely government-financed but relying in part on private funds and having above-average internal autonomy. These include the Karolinska Institute in Stockholm and the various Max Planck Institutes in Germany.

Both governmental and private research institutes can be subdivided into mission-oriented or general. A mission-oriented medical research institute would have as its corporate goal the solution of a specific disease problem. Most countries have private and/or governmental cancer research institutes; many have institutes devoted to other specific important medical areas such as heart research, arthritis, child health. A general institute, such as 'Mill Hill' or the Rockefeller, chooses its areas of research endeavour in less specific fashion, the particular research interests of the director and his senior staff at any given time being the main determining factors. The distinction is not as clear-cut as it seems, for two reasons. First, it is very difficult to pre-judge what type of research will influence eventual treatment of a disease such as cancer or coronary occlusion, so that most mission-oriented institutes rightly maintain a permissive stance towards basic science. Secondly, in all institutes of real quality, the individual investigator retains considerable freedom; in my experience there is little categorical difference between workers in the two types of institutes, so that through individual free choice the dividing line becomes blurred.

A new type of research institute has emerged recently, which is full of fascination and promise. It is the supra-national or multi-national research institute. Examples are CERN (Centre Européen de Recherches Néucleaires), IARC (International Agency for Research on Cancer) and the planned EMBO (European Molecular Biology Organization) institute. In these, both staffing and financing are international, and great emphasis is placed on collaborative projects and teamwork. Of course, basic science is already a highly international affair, but formal recognition of the role of science as a unifying world force by the creation of these bodies can do only good.

## Characteristic advantages and disadvantages of research institutes

It is clear from the above description that medical research institutes are a heterogeneous collection. However, some common characteristics pertain to all. Obviously the most important is that the staff are engaged and paid solely to do medical research. They have no major 'teaching load'. Usually, their undergraduate teaching commitments are confined to a few lectures given by invitation at friendly universities. In many cases, however, there is a substantial commitment of time to graduate education. At the local level, many research institutes maintain a university affiliation which allows them to accept candidates for advanced degrees, such as the Ph. D. These graduate students perform valuable research but also require rigorous teaching and supervision. At the national and international level, research leaders from institutes are widely involved in addressing congresses and meetings, thus contributing to post-graduate teaching in the widest sense. I mention this type of teaching spin-off from research institutes because it is not widely appreciated and because the 'ivory tower' image of the man in a research institute is often overdone. Nevertheless, the absence of a substantial teaching commitment is one of the biggest differences between the life of an institute worker and his University counterpart. Another, allied difference is that the full-time researcher tends to be less involved in committee work and administration than the University man, as the affairs of the latter, larger organization tend to be more complex and varied. This difference applies only to intramural committees; most prominent research institute workers take at least their fair share of the work on expert government committees and in running scientific societies and journals. With all these considerations in mind, one could sum up by saying that the institute worker will have 70–80% of his time for research as opposed to 30–50% of his time in the case of the typical university lecturer, though in the latter category exceptions in either direction will occur.

This advantage for research in favour of the institute is counter balanced by some disadvantages, the importance of which varies greatly from institution to institution. One potential problem is that of isolation. The University man rubs shoulders daily with many students, and at less frequent intervals will have professional or semi-social contacts with fellow academics in the humanities, social sciences and physical sciences. The research institute man will tend far more to be professionally surrounded by those of his own ilk. The problem is worst in small, highly-specialized institutes geographically remote from other centres of learning. Isolation can also take the form of a tendency for a relatively small and stable staff to grow to think alike and to reinforce one another's intellectual conservatism. The strongest counter balance to such trends and one which I have found extremely effective in my own institution, is to maintain a steady flow through an institute of gifted younger workers from other centres or even countries. We shall have much to say in chapter 5 about this uniquely important category comprising graduate students, post-doctoral fellows and junior staff members. These individuals, attached to an institute for periods of one to four years, can make all the difference to the level of intellectual excitement pervading it. Altogether, it is difficult to overestimate the influence of the young in research, with their capacity to challenge set ideas, their drive and boldness. Here the University man enjoys an advantage over many of his institute colleagues. Another feature is that teaching, often referred to as a 'load', can also readily be a joy and solace. In the lives of all research men there are difficult, dull patches when experiments are not going well and creativity seems at a low ebb. In the case of the University man, the distress caused by such periods is leavened by the continuation of his less fluctuating contribution to education. The lecturer also has the great joy of first identification of the exceptionally gifted newcomer, and rightly takes pride in the possibility of influencing him to the good at an impressionable stage of development.

At a level more remote from the individual worker, a subtle difficulty faces research institutes, particularly private ones. Universities perform a readily visible social function, and though their level of affluence will vary to a certain extent with political changes, most enjoy reasonable financial stability. The social contribution of a pure research institute is much more intangible, and may in fact be invisible to those unfamiliar with the nexus-progression of human scientific knowledge analyzed in Chapter 1. In a real sense, research institutes are a glory but also a luxury. If they run into hard times, it is difficult to make a social or political issue out of this. In general, an institute's financial situation is more dependent on current economic conditions, government policy and short-range productivity of research staff than is that of a University.

Below, we will entertain some criticisms of university-based and industry-based researchers, so the institute man should not be made to appear a paragon. People are people, in all walks of life, and laziness and incompetence are frequent human traits. A research institute is in many ways an ideal haven for a reasonably smart person who has given up the struggle for excellence or has run out of steam. In general, freedom of personal movement and a general permissiveness with regard to hours of work is present; objective criteria of lack of productivity are less tangible than in industry; and straight forward sackings are quite rare. Thus, nearly all Institutes have a proportion of relative 'dead weight'. Part of the function of a director is to minimize this proportion and to motivate the less able or willing workers into assuming duties under someone else's supervision. A problem of somewhat different complexion is that of the research man who in his youth was very good, who is still a willing and conscientious worker, but who is no longer having sufficiently original ideas, or whose field has become overworked and tedious. This problem can only be attacked by persuading the person to move into an entirely new area of work, initially with guidance from someone who may be his junior. I have seen several encouraging revivals of careers in men with sufficient humility to allow this approach.

**Life in a typical medical research institute**

From the foregoing, it will be clear that most of the disadvantages outlined for research institutes are not too difficult to overcome. They remain the ideal organization in which to perform medical research. Although I have said that many different types of medical research institute exist, it may nevertheless be helpful to describe my own institute, which in many respects is typical. A history of the Walter and Eliza Hall Institute of Medical Research has been published by my predecessor, Sir Macfarlane Burnet, and the reader is referred to this for details of structure and financing. The Hall Institute comprises some 160 people, putting it in the medium-sized category by world standards, though it is the largest institute of its kind in Australia. Its main subject area is immunology, the study of the body's lymphocyte cells in both health and disease. However, quite a number of other related and unrelated research efforts occupy about 40% of the scene, including projects in cancer research, embryology, bio-medical computation and genetics. Research policy is dictated by the director, and his senior staff. In this instance, the key group is small, consisting of only 6 people, each in charge of an independent unit. The unit heads are expected to be internationally-known leaders of research. Each has full autonomy in directing his programme and almost full discretion on questions such as numbers and nature of his staff, subject always to his ability to raise the necessary grant support through governmental agencies or private foundations. The director has responsibility for ensuring that the training and skills of his unit heads are diverse and complementary, so that broad institutional research goals can be espoused and achieved. He can also exert influence to encourage inter-unit collaboration, allowing important problems to be attacked by people of diverse backgrounds, and lending a multi-disciplinary flavour to the institute's effort. Indeed, teamwork seems to be one of the key requirements towards major achievements in the biosciences today. Each unit, in turn, will consist of six to ten scientists and a number of technicians. Depending on their rank and experience, these scientists again will have a considerable degree of scientific autonomy, although the subject areas of their research must mesh with the long-range goals of the unit head. In all, there are some fifty scientists in the institute, and an equal number of technicians either in laboratories or in centralized scientific services. The remainder of the staff is made up of administrative, secretarial, animal-care and other ancillary personnel.

The amount of time that each of the scientists spends actually physically manipulating experimental material at the laboratory bench will vary inversely with his seniority. A graduate student or post-doctoral fellow will spend up to 90% of his official working time at the bench. He has no duties or responsibilities other than his research project. Of course, he is expected to read the scientific literature, but is encouraged to do this on evenings or week-ends. Some time will go into planning experiments, discussions with supervisors, and preparation of scientific talks or papers, but essentially the 'bench' is his life. In contrast, a unit head must perforce spend much more time on discussion, supervision, planning, integrating, writing and cajoling his collaborators towards certain directions. Despite this, it is a common experience that those supervisors who divorce themselves altogether from the bench lose much of their effectiveness within a few years. I, myself, try to retain 50% of my time for straight laboratory work. Clearly, the situation of staff scientists between these extremes of seniority will be intermediate.

Life in a research institute is thus a blend of technical manipulation, thought and discussion, teaching and learning, full of fascination and variety. An extra complexity arises in the case of clinical research organizations, where the staff have responsibilities not only for research but also for patient care. For example, one of our six units is a clinical research unit, and the unit head is a senior physician in the Royal Melbourne Hospital, with full responsibility for the care of both inpatients and outpatients. Several of his staff also help care for the sick, so naturally the time available for the laboratory bench is reduced. We have found it most interesting and useful to create an interface between 'ivory tower' and practical bedside medicine within the one organization. Though both pure science and clinical medicine require intelligence, knowledge and judgement, there are many differences in approach. In his scientific work, a man must remain sceptical, cool, objective and can frequently afford the luxury of fence-sitting. In his clinical investigational work, the same applies to the ward doctor, but he must in some way try to balance his scientific objectivity with decisiveness, and sufficient human warmth and strength to help his patient. In particular he must treat his patient with what he *believes* to be the best remedies, frequently in the absence of the sort of rigorous proof of superiority that the scientific side of his make-up may demand. The intellectual interactions between clinicians and pure scientists, especially in the context of discussions on individual patients, are often of surprising value to all parties. There is much mutual learning, both as regards actual problems and remote research goals. While not relevant to every specialized medical research institute, the presence of a clinical unit can thus be a most salutary feature. It certainly reminds the basic scientist that a wealth of problems of direct human importance remain to be tackled, thus helping to 'keep his feet on the ground'. In an era where young people are increasingly concerned about the social relevance of human endeavours, the symbolic value of clinical-scientific interactions is especially great.

We will return to a consideration of clinical research in a more practical way after the section dealing with research in the pharmaceutical industry.

We can summarize the ideals towards which the Hall Institute is striving in terms of its organizational framework. These include a major world impact in immunology, cancer research and related areas through a broad team effort; a constant search for new research areas and goals of importance; a vigorous flow through the institute of young scientists from many countries; close, collegial links with affiliated university and hospital; activity of our scientists on many teaching fronts, particularly at the international level; effective collaboration between scientists and groups, and between clinical and non-clinical arms; and maximum job satisfaction for staff, both junior and senior. No institutional framework, however superb, can guarantee what all researchers agree to be the acme of scientific achievement, namely the discovery of some very basic new fact or principle which alters in a major way the history of a scientific field. Such 'breakthroughs' do exist, but are rare, and depend on individual genius. It is reassuring to note that when they do occur, it is most frequently by members of organizations that are at or near the top in their 'conventional' scientific research.

## Pure and applied research in medical research institutes

The example I have chosen so far is of an institute which engages in both pure and applied research. In fact, many institutes, the name of which implies a commitment only to applied research, are in a similar position. A cancer research institute would normally contain a large component of pure research on cell function and chemistry, and would also have applied laboratories investigating practical cancer problems (such as a search for better anti-cancer drugs). There are, of course, many institutes which are 'all pure' or 'all applied'. The Salk Institute in California is a good example of a first-rate pure biological research institute with no clinical arm. It is already evident that some of their 'pure science' discoveries will have clinical relevance eventually. The British Medical Research Council has just built an 'applied' counterpart of their world-famous 'pure' Institute (Mill Hill). This centre will be almost entirely devoted to *clinical* science, though naturally much laboratory work will go on. Therefore, it is clearly inadvisable to make value judgements about which kind of Institute is most important. Each has its place, and through this healthy diversity, medical science as a whole progresses.

**Medical research in universities**

Through traditions dating back many centuries, universities are expected not only to preserve and dispense knowledge, but also to create it. The need for universities to do research has never been in any doubt. However, in the past two decades, an increasing controversy has arisen about the relative importance of research and teaching in universities. Much public reaction has implied that the socially-necessary teaching duties have been neglected because of over-emphasis on socially-unnecessary research. The issue is a complex one, and full treatment is outside the scope of this book. However my belief is that, in the sciences at least, research and teaching are inextricably linked, and I suspect that the same holds true in the humanities, though perhaps to a lesser degree. The point will be developed in Chapter 7; here I wish to describe the present status of medical research in universities, and some of the problems and challenges that the university researcher faces.

The 'teaching load' of a university lecturer in a medical or biological subject varies enormously from country to country and institution to institution. In some of the top United States medical schools such as Harvard or Stanford, the staff:student ratio is so high that the number of required teaching hours is quite small and the overall situation of many staff members little different from that of his institute counterpart. In many less privileged centres – and the problem is world-wide – the staff:student ratio is so low that teaching absorbs virtually all the available time and attempts at research become a mere pretence. However, the majority of universities find themselves in an intermediate position, as do a *minority* of individuals in the two extremes cited. How do such universities cope with the problem?

To a greater extent than is the case in research institutes, the answer lies with individuals. At the beginning of his career, the university instructor or junior lecturer is chosen mainly because of his research promise. Moreover, continued research productivity is an important factor in his rate of promotion. However, in most universities there occurs a very natural 'free-market' development of load distribution between teaching and research. A few individuals show outstanding research ability. Such a person gradually builds up a substantial group around him; he breezes through his set lectures and delegates the more time-consuming demonstrating duties to graduate students. Frequently his colleagues recognize the special gift and shield him from the less interesting teaching chores. Other lecturers may be less gifted for research but find themselves to be effective, dedicated teachers. Gradually, they lighten their research programmes or leave more and more of the bench work to students. Their drive goes into education, their satisfaction comes from student recognition. Colleagues realize the nature of such a man's gifts and inclinations, and promotion, though surely slower, will come on the basis of excellence in teaching. Thus, particularly in larger departments, there is the possibility of considerable variation in the research to teaching ratio. Undoubtedly my university colleagues will regard the above as an oversimplification, and I do not intend my analysis to imply the absence of a problem. It *is* harder for the University man to find adequate time for research, particularly when experiments require large blocks of continuous, uninterrupted time. Moreover, while biology is advancing so rapidly, it is difficult to keep up. A good one hour lecture may require many hours to prepare, especially as lecturers must frequently cover aspects of a field in which they themselves are not acknowledged experts. The University man can only compete in research at world level after extra effort and struggle; yet I believe it vitally important for him to win that struggle and to remain in research. The reasons for this will emerge in Chapter 7.

This brings us to the problem of administration in universities. For the head of a department, these are large and difficult to resolve. A university is different from an industrial concern of equivalent size, where authority flows according to well-defined, accepted patterns. In fact, universities are collections of a hundred or more fiefdoms, with each department chairman claiming pre-eminence in his particular field, and hence equality. In turn, he will have on his staff experts in various branches of learning, each with a considerable self-esteem. In short, academics tend to be *prima donnas*. Moreover, the problems which arise frequently cannot readily be resolved by non-experts. Finally, university dons are usually liberals and strong advocates of democratic processes and individual rights. Most of this is good; much of it inevitable; but it *does* add up to an administrative nightmare. Long periods of academic time are used up in committee meetings where issues are discussed endlessly and frequently circularly. I wonder whether most student activists realize how many man-hours go into assessing the validity of student demands, or how conscientiously the special pleadings of a failed student are judged? A disproportionate fraction of this kind of work falls on department heads, not to mention their intra-departmental duties in curriculum formulation, grant administration and personnel work. Little wonder, then, that most university department chairmen have virtually no time for research. In fact, in the United States the situation has created a crisis, because the more gifted professors simply do not want to take chairmanships. In Great Britain, Europe and Australia, the extra power and prestige of being the head still draws the best men into the job, but frequently the job destroys the man. No easy solution has yet been found. Rotating chairmanships represent one approach, appointment of experienced administrators as assistants to the chairman another. Some professors disengage entirely from the wider problems of the university and guard their research time in that way. Others survive through 90-hour work weeks. A few are very gifted at delegation, which may represent the best available solution. In all, the dilemma of the multiple duties of the University department chairman remains one of major proportions.

The age of competitiveness and teamwork in discovery has uncovered another disadvantage suffered by the university researcher. Major medical subjects such as physiology or microbiology are by now so large that they are virtually an amalgam of sub-specialities. A virologist with molecular biologic leanings would have little in common with an expert in the taxonomy of the fungal species which produce antibiotics, yet both are microbiologists. Most department chairmen feel that for teaching to be optimal, they must have on their staff experts in numerous sub-specialities. This may militate against teamwork in research and leave the university man handicapped *vis a vis* his institute counterpart, as in specialized institutes, staff are chosen on the basis of like and complementary interests.

Much of the above sounds pessimistic with respect to university medical research, and in effect one has the feeling that over the last twenty years the ratio of truly important work coming out of institutes rather than universities has definitely increased. Nevertheless highly distinguished contributions continue to be made in universities despite the obstacles. I count myself a strong advocate of research in universities, chiefly because I cannot see how the universities could continue their main mission of undergraduate and postgraduate education without a strong internal research base. The point is subtle, but I believe it to be so important that I shall devote the whole of Chapter 7 to it and related issues.

## Competitiveness in research

Much of the controversy around university medical research centres around the concept of competitiveness. The opponents of research in universities stress that the obstacles outlined above are such as to render the university man unable to compete with the institute worker. With such vast masses of ignorance remaining, why should there be any question of competing? Why could not every senior man pursue his own individual, unique line of investigation at his own pace? One is frequently asked about duplication of research effort. Why is it that important discoveries are frequently made independently and virtually simultaneously by two or three groups? Could not some central authority avoid wasteful duplication?

These questions are real and important, yet I feel certain that ninety-nine per cent of researchers would instantly reply that competitiveness and duplication are an inevitable and even useful part of the modern science picture. The reasons are many and complex. The total number of researchers is now very large and communication is effective, thus the statistical chance of a perceived duplication is raised. While the totality of ignorance is immense, the number of ways of approaching major problems is finite and limited by technological factors. Moreover, though myriads of problems of detail abound, the number of definable, truly important research issues in any one area is much smaller. Finally, independent confirmation of a finding by another worker or group is an essential part of the progress of science.

These are clear and defensible considerations, and I would be the first to affirm the importance of a continued 'free market' approach to research organization. Bureaucratic control of a creative exercise simply does not work. On the other hand, I believe there is a valid area for concern with respect to work that is little more than a 're-hash' of some past discovery. We have discussed bandwagons already, and I believe the cause of science as a whole would be well served if granting bodies took a sterner stance against research projects that are technically competent but essentially unoriginal. This would force the less prominent workers to think a little harder. He would espouse less ambitious but more individualistic research goals, rather than hop on to the bandwagon and achieve reflected glory from 'me, too' type experiments. The university man, if isolated or part of a very small group, can still do most useful research in a restricted, less glamorous area; but if he seeks to compete for a discovery also being sought by larger, prominent, well-funded institutional groups, he is likely to be swamped.

## Further Inter-relationships between Pure and Applied Research, and between research and development

In a broad sense, it is therefore evident that no clear distinction can be made between the research done in institutes and that in universities, with respect to its nature and its goals. These academic institutions are best fitted to contribute basic new knowledge in the health sciences. There remains, then, the question of how this knowledge is to be applied to practical problems. In medical research, the issue is how a new insight into the workings of a biological system or the nature of a specific disease process can be translated into a tablet, an injection or an operation that can prevent or cure an illness. This means applied research. Next, there will arise problems related to scaling up; if a drug or a vaccine is a real advance, how to make enough of it to provide a million doses, of adequate standards of safety and effectiveness, and how to determine that one person in 100,000 will not have an adverse reaction? This represents the development phase of the project.

I believe the public gravely underestimates the difficulty of the applied research and development phases, and I fear many academics undervalue the contribution made by workers in these fields. I think the time is ripe for a major reappraisal which takes cognisance both of the human value and the inherent intellectual interest and challenge of applied research and development. If university academics could imbue their students with a more positive image of 'practical' research, the placement of Ph. D. graduates would be less of a problem, the quality of applied research would improve, and the public image of science would gradually change to the better. As it is, there does exist somewhat of an image – or prestige-gap between the industrial scientist and the academic in medical research. In view of the immense impact of industry-based research in the development of a physician's therapeutic armamenterium, this is really unwarranted.

We must now look in detail at the great 'third world' in medical research, namely the research divisions of the large pharmaceutical manufacturers. It is a world that is poorly understood and much maligned by workers in the other two, and some (but only some) of the criticism is deserved. We shall approach our analysis first by asking what industry-based research does; then how it does it; and finally how these patterns might be improved.

## Goals and achievements of research within the pharmaceutical industry

Human motivations are mixed, and this is true as much for institutions as it is for individuals. Thus the research division of a large pharmaceutical manufacturing concern will have as its central goal the discovery and testing of new and effective drugs that can then be developed and marketed by the company. One motive and consideration will be financial profit;

another humanitarian concern; another corporate or individual prestige; another intellectual curiosity and fascination. It is too facile to pretend that the profit motive is the only one, but quite stupid to pretend that it does not exist. Interestingly, the free enterprise system works very effectively in the development of new drugs. Sir Derrick Dunlop, Britain's foremost authority on therapeutics, is on record as saying that of the 50 most valuable drugs in existence, not a single one has come from a communist country. So the dominant concern of industry research is to find new drugs for profit. However, the other concerns are of sufficient importance to ensure that industrial researchers are drawn into quite a few pure research endeavours. It is simply the 'mix' of pure versus applied that is slanted more heavily in the latter direction.

These corporate goals can best be understood by concrete examples. Let us look at the field of antibiotics. In 1929, Alexander Fleming first noted that the common bread-mold, *Penicillium notatum*, manufactured a substance which powerfully inhibited the growth of bacteria. Ten years later Howard Florey and Ernst Chain set about a systematic chemical approach to the purification of the active principle, penicillin. Their efforts culminated in the availability of a very small amount of material for clinical use, sufficient to show that penicillin was indeed a miracle drug. Florey himself persuaded the American drug industry to set up the large-scale fermentations necessary for bulk production, and some very fundamental contributions, such as the use of submerged cultures, were made by industry researchers. Therefore the U.S. pharmaceutical manufacturers deserve a good proportion of the credit for the wide availability of penicillin in World War II theatres. After the war, large programmes were started in many firms to find and produce new antibiotics. The principle that molds could produce antibacterials had been established as the result of 'pure' research. It stood to reason that other molds would make other antibiotics, and the patient search involved could be regarded as 'applied' research. Streptomycin, the first antibiotic with activity in tuberculosis, was in fact discovered by Waksman, an academic. However, the great bulk of other antibiotics, many of them crucially important to modern therapeutics, were discovered by the drug industry. A broadly similar tale could be told for poliomyelitis vaccine. John Enders and colleagues learnt that the polio virus could be grown in cultures of living monkey cells. Jonas Salk did marvellous development work in learning how to kill the virus without destroying its capacity to immunize, and in testing vaccine potency in experimental animals. It took big industry, however, to do the scaling up necessary for the resolution of the great human problem.

These examples illustrate situations where the industry's contribution was a reasonably predictable one, given the original breakthrough. There are, however, many examples where the whole 'head of power' for major therapeutic advances has come from industry. Take, for example, the revolution in mental health that has taken place over the last fifteen years. While the incidence of psychotic disorders is certainly no less, the outlook for the psychotic patient is vastly improved. This is reflected by a much shorter length of stay in mental asylums, a substantial cure rate and even complete rehabilitation of patients thought to be quite beyond help. The story of how this all started is worth telling. Anti-histamine pills have been on the market for many years, and are of use in certain allergies like hay fever. However, as many readers will heartily agree, these pills make one very sleepy. In 1951, scientists at a French pharmaceutical house called Rhone Poulenc got the bright idea of seeing whether this undesirable side effect could be turned to good use. They were looking for something that would be an aid to the induction of anesthesia, and, to cut a long story short, they synthesized an antihistamine-like drug, called chlorpromazine, and carried out the first clinical investigations with it in 1952. It soon became apparent that this agent was indeed very useful in reducing agitation before an operation, in tranquillizing people, if you will, and it was a useful anaesthetic aid. This tranquillizing action was unexpectedly strong, so naturally the drug was soon tried in acutely disturbed mental patients. It was found to be extremely effective in a wide variety of psychiatric states, including schizophrenia and the agitated phase of manic-depressive psychosis. And so, the modern era of drug treatment of mental disease was born out of an accident, the fact that antihistaminics make you sleepy. Drug-industry researchers naturally now began to look amongst the chemical relatives of chlorpromazine for new and better drugs, and the yield has been phenomenal. In 1957 came imipramine, which is now a widely used and very effective drug against severe depression. Another spin-off, less useful albeit more profitable, has been the development of the so-called minor tranquillizers, Librium, Miltown and the like, which are said to relieve anxiety in normal or mildly neurotic people. The popular supposition that such agents are able to allay ordinary everyday worries has been widely disputed. In any case, this is not our primary concern. The thing I want to stress is that the pharmaceutical industry has played a key initiating and continuing role in this line of research.

It is therefore clear that the industry worker must involve himself deeply in modern research trends. He must be ever alert to these basic findings most likely to yield practical pay-off in the short to medium term. He must take over where the basic researcher chooses to leave off, and must overlap with him. In my own field of immunology the drug industry is actively involved in much research that is still 'fairly pure' but that could blossom into marketable products within five years. There are, in fact, many projects where academic and industry researcher collaborate actively with mutual benefit. There is no *a priori* reason why a career in drug research should not be fascinating and fulfilling.

## Organization of research in the pharmaceutical industry

The research divisions of major pharmaceutical firms have much in common with medical research institutes. It is common industry practice to spend ten per cent of world sales, or a sum roughly equal to net profit, on research. This means huge budgets, say $US 20 to 50 million, for the larger corporations. In many cases, nearly all of this is spent in one large institution built close to the firm's headquarters. There tends to be much less geographic fragmentation of research than of production facilities. The large, centralized research division may employ some hundreds of Ph. D. and M.D. graduates and an equal number of ancillary personnel. In size, many are much larger than famous national research institutes.

Organizationally, there are some big differences from research institutes. Much of the difference stems from necessary commercial considerations. While industry scientists are encouraged to publish their basic science findings in the open literature, it is clear that some degree of secrecy must, for patent purposes, surround early stages of discoveries of commercial value. Moreover, a good portion of the work of an industry researcher, such as routine screening of large numbers of compounds for a particular drug effect, or extensive testing of a new product for possible toxicity, is essentially poor material for publication purposes. Therefore, the 'routine' work of the industry man is often not published. Publication record is the biggest single factor in defining a research man's status. Thus, the less gifted industry worker may gradually sink from the view of his colleagues in academe. Unless he belongs to the outstanding few, or unless he 'cracks' a big discovery, his statistical chances of returning to academe diminish progressively with time. The result is a greater degree of job stability in the industry as opposed to the academic community. Shifting from firm to firm does occur, but much less frequently than from university to university. This results in a greater potential for 'inbreeding' and a higher median age for staff than is the case in most universities. One way or another, a certain isolation from the mainstream of research in the 'other two worlds' is an ever-present danger. This is actively combatted by the better firms. These insist that their researchers keep up their contacts with their specialist learned societies, present papers at meetings, and so forth. They also invite visiting lecturers and consultants to interact with the industry scientists. Nevertheless, it is my impression that most academics make little allowance for the special circumstances pertaining to drug firm research, and tend to 'look down' a little on the man who works for industry. Any of my colleagues could quickly point to outstanding exceptions, men of the highest academic rank who work for drug firms, names who grace the programmes of the most erudite meetings, and so forth. However, in their heart of hearts they would grudgingly agree that a certain 'status gap' does exist for the *average* pharmaceutical industry scientist as opposed to the *average* academic.

There is a certain vicious cycle element in this situation. The status gap may itself be a factor in preventing the best young graduates from going into industry; the man of lesser quality who accordingly takes the industry job may hold it a very long time; and so forth. Perhaps an unexpected benefit will flow from the current fiscal cut-backs in research in the United States, in that this cycle could be broken.

Another organizational difference between the industrial and the academic research scene is that in the former there exists a substantial managerial class forming a link between bench scientist and corporate management. These research managers are scientists, but tend to become entirely separated from the bench and involved in both straight administration and corporate politics. In general, their degree of power over the bench scientist is greater than that of department chairman over faculty member; in the latter case, there is always the possibility of going and getting an outside grant. Yet, their level of understanding of experimental detail may be slight. This presents frequent problems in the industry.

## Improvements possible in drug research

One of the worst features of research in the drug industry is the work which needs to be done to make and test products which are only marginally different from existing ones. As soon as a real therapeutic advance occurs, there is a great temptation for a competitor to come along with a drug differing slightly in chemical composition which can then be marketed without patent infringement. This kind of work is mentally stultifying and, with rare exceptions, of no benefit to mankind. A possible answer would be a certain degree of voluntary rationalization of product lines within the industry. I fear, however, that to a degree this wastefulness is built into the system, and part of the price we have to pay for the free market framework. Of course, the medical profession could play a greater role in not prescribing drugs which purport to be new but are really only minor variants of existing satisfactory products.

I should also like to see a freer exchange of views and information between the industrial and academic worlds. Industry could be a little less sensitive about patent protection for research and academics a little more generous in recognition of their industry colleagues. A somewhat more dynamic staffing policy by industry, with greater emphasis on continued individual productivity (in the scientific sense) would also help. In this way, the 'third world' could be brought more into the mainstream of medical science. Finally, it would help if industrial research managers could maintain closer contacts with the bench, and if a pattern of organization could develop whereby the more gifted scientists could build up power and prestige within a company while still heavily engaged in research.

## Clinical testing of drugs

There eventually comes a time in the progress of research when a new drug must go into man for the first time. This is preceded by an interval of many months or even years of toxicity testing in a variety of animal species, frequently including monkeys and chimpanzees. As part of such testing, doses greatly in excess of the necessary therapeutic dose are given, and the animals are carefully examined from every possible biochemical and physiological viewpoint to determine what toxic 'side effects' do show up. Obviously, the best drugs are those which show a high 'therapeutic ratio', i.e. where the dose which produces undesirable side effects is much larger than that which is needed for effective disease treatment. Nevertheless, many drugs do show unpleasant side effects at relatively low dose, and the physician must use judgement to balance the good versus the harm. Many side effects are predictable from the animal work; some do not show up until clinical trial. The first occasion that a drug goes into man is always an occasion of some risk, but the animal research and previous work on related drugs ensures that this is usually a minimal one. Enormous publicity was rightly given to the thalidomide disaster, where a sedative drug influenced limb development in human embryos. This should not obscure the fact that hundreds of new drugs have been tested and introduced without major disasters, and that many more have never reached the market because animal or very preliminary human work have shown up toxicity.

In the United States, extensive use is made of prisoners as volunteers for drug testing. The prisoner who collaborates with a pharmaceutical firm in

UNIVERSITY OF BRISTOL MEDICINE

a research project has a portion of his sentence remitted. This type of volunteer is not favoured in most other countries, where it is more usual to give the initial doses of a new compound to a small number of patients, who are, of course, informed that they are receiving a new drug and who volunteer to take the risk. The next phase of drug testing is usually a collaboration between industry and academics. The firm that believes it has a new product persuades a number of highly regarded clinical researchers in hospitals or universities to compare the effectiveness of the new product with whatever may be the standard treatment. It goes without saying that in many countries strict legislation exists to cover the phase of clinical testing. In the United States, for example, the Food and Drug Authority is charged with this responsibility, and getting a new drug approved for clinical testing is a long and arduous process. It has been estimated that the time gap between a 'breakthrough' in the industrial research laboratory, and the eventual availability on prescription of the drug that finally results, now averages seven years! This highlights the fact, perhaps not known to many people, that clinical testing is not undertaken lightly. Moreover, the design of clinical trials of new drugs follows rigid statistical criteria. A favourite approach is the 'double-blind, controlled trial', in which every second patient with a particular disease gets the new drug, and every other patient an identical-looking tablet or capsule, which however contains either no drug or else some old, established remedy. In such trials, neither the doctor nor the patient knows which person is receiving the real tablet and which the 'dummy'. Thus psychological factors are minimized. The code is broken after an interval usually pre-determined before the trial starts by statistical consultants.

One could write much more on techniques of drug testing and evaluation, which is indeed a major facet of clinical research. The key thing to note is the enormous contrast between the vast scientific effort involved in establishing a real medical advance; and the incredible gullibility of many sick people when it comes to 'quack' remedies. Medical science frequently deliberates for years about the definitive role of a drug in treatment, yet the lay person in distress will clutch at straws and thereby encourage the unsavoury crowd of cancer quacks and other self-styled experts who parasitize human misery.

*Further reading*

Bernal, J. D. *The Social Function of Science*. George Routledge and Sons Ltd, London (1939).

Burnet, F. M. *Walter and Eliza Hall Institute 1915–1965*. Melbourne University Press

(1971).
Cockcroft, J. D. ed., *The Organization of Research Establishments*. Cambridge University Press (1965).
Cotgrove S. and Box, S. *Science, Industry and Society*. George Allen and Unwin Ltd, London (1970).
Kaplan, N. ed., *Science and Society*. Rand McNally and Co. Chicago (1965).
Snow, C. P. *Public Affairs*. Macmillan, London (1971).

# 4

# The medical scientist: attributes, aspirations, motivations, interactions

*'The creative act is alike in art and in science, but it cannot be identical; there must be a difference as well as a likeness. For example, the artist in his creation surely has open to him a dimension of freedom which is closed to the scientist'.* J. Bronowski

There is a substantial gap between the image of the medical scientist that most people carry in their mind and the actuality of his personality, his hopes and his interactions with colleagues and society. From what we have already considered, it will be clear that the army of medical researchers is now very large and embraces a heterogeneous group of people. Nevertheless, there are a sufficient number of common characteristics to make an attempted analysis worthwhile. As a prelude, it is worth stating that the central prerequisite for major progress in science is a judicious mixture of imagination and discipline. The former is at least as important as in the arts or the humanities, and the latter even more so, because good science requires a great degree of repetition of effort.

The stock image that the layman has of a medical researcher represents a singularly idealized version. The layman endows us with great dedication, selfless devotion, profound commitment to the relief of suffering. He has in mind a tall, thin, bookish man with spectacles; stethoscope hanging from the pocket of a threadbare white coat; slaving away in the laboratory night and day while the world rolls by. This vision was inaccurate even in Pasteur's time, and is even more so today. Medical research is a profession, an acknowledged career alternative for both medical and science students when they consider their future on graduation. As such, it will draw into its orbit people not so very different from those entering other professions. It is naive to believe that practical and selfish considerations, such as salary, promotional opportunities and quality of life do not influence a person's choice of a research career. Unquestionably a tinge of idealism exists and one drawing force is the possibility of doing something of major benefit for mankind as a whole. In general, young academics do have an above-average degree of social consciousness. However, this is far from the whole story.

Our study of the human aspects of the medical scientist can begin by a look at the qualities of mind and spirit that go into the making of a good researcher. Then we can look in more detail at his real motivating forces, and the kinds of structures that the 'peer group' creates to aid interactions between scientists.

## Qualities needed in a research worker

Few fields of decision-making are as complex and as uncertain as the prospective assessment of human creativity. After fifteen intensive years in medical research, I still make big mistakes in choosing new staff. The three qualities which appear most desirable are analytical ability, originality and drive.

By analytical ability I mean a capacity to think in abstract terms, and both a liking for and a competence in problem-solving. This is the kind of 'intelligence' that will give a pupil good marks in mathematics or physics. The budding scientist usually has far less difficulty than other people in recognizing why a fairly detailed and specialized research experiment appearing trivial on first inspection, may be a proper concern of a highly-paid research group. He will see the problem as a model relevant to a larger principle, and will enjoy the challenge of grappling with its difficulties. Together with power for abstraction will go a critical faculty. This means an ability to sift evidence and a tendency to challenge established beliefs; most potential research recruits like to examine their society in this way and incidentally make stern and perceptive critics of their scientific mentors! This broad heading of analytical intelligence is reflected to a certain degree in good performance at examinations. However, while there will be a broad, general correlation between high school and undergraduate examination performance and eventual research ability, there are numerous exceptions in both directions. Brilliant youngsters whose student record is studded with prizes may fail in research because their good memory and keen brain does not make up for a lack of originality. Conversely, poor students may end up as good researchers because of a certain dreamy quality that can flower later. In an imperfect world, good grades are probably still the best predicitive guides out of an uncertain lot available.

Originality is a quality more difficult to define. It is a blend of intuition and unconventionality; an ability to make new syntheses of facts and ideas that previously seemed unconnected. Original research ideas frequently come without conscious volition – be it under the shower or during a vigorous exchange of views with a colleague – and one is tempted to look for words like inspiration or creative insight to describe their occurrence. Some authors have compared the quality of originality in research to the creative act of the composer or the artist. Sir Peter Medawar has found himself puzzled about the mainsprings of originality and has written a fascinating book on the subject (see reading list). It is, of course, possible to do effective research without much originality, by assiduous exploration of lines of work opened up through the originality of others. This can be satisfying and worthwhile. As few people enter research without a higher than normal analytic intelligence, however, the presence of originality frequently becomes a discriminating feature between the excellent and the merely competent researcher.

There is an interesting paradox to be resolved concerning critical analytic ability versus originality in research. In most original research discoveries as they first emerge, there is a sufficient element of doubt and tentativeness to give scope to a stern critic; it is relatively easy for an intelligent man to pick holes in the incomplete but truly new discovery, and to conclude that it is not worth worrying about until more evidence comes forward to confirm it. Similarly, critical analysis can usually find fault in design of an original experiment yet to be performed. There are some scientists who are so critical that they talk themselves out of most experiments that they conceive! The overly critical, highly intelligent but unoriginal scientist can become a negative force in research. There is a need to strike a balance, to temper critical objectivity with creative enthusiasm, and to take a few risks.

The third quality, that of drive, will certainly not have occurred to most lay readers, yet it is very important. There is much tedious routine in both the performance and the recording of research. Experiments have to be repeated a number of times; sophisticated techniques, exciting when first developed, soon become routine; results, when confirmed must be written up and annotated, with due deference to the stylized and somewhat ponderous language of formal scientific papers. All of this consumes energy. Also, we have noted that research in most fields has become competitive. There is no virtue in being the *second* person to make a discovery. Often, the first will be not necessarily the more intelligent worker but the one with more drive, initiative and organizational skill. I know quite a number of scientists with adequate intelligence and originality who totally lack 'killer instinct'. They make valuable members of institutes in positions of lesser responsibility, and can become well-liked members of the peer group, but it is not often that they make really fundamental contributions. With the rare exception of the dreamy near-genius, who fortunately still exists in modern science, the research leader of today is a driving man, 'aggressive' in the American sense of the word, and I suspect the reader would be surprised at how similar some of his gifts are to those of the successful executive. However, it is unusual for a scientist to have the executive's flair for communication. Indeed, many scientists with otherwise well-integrated personalities are poor communicators, even in a strictly technical setting. This is a noteworthy factor adding to the tedium of many scientific meetings!

**Selection of research staff**

It is the experience of most research administrators that it is very difficult to predict which individual will make a good scientist before that individual has been placed in an actual operational setting in the laboratory. The problem is worse for M.D. than for Ph.D. graduates. The Ph.D. has already got three to four years of laboratory involvement 'under his belt' when he gets his degree, and it should be reasonably clear by then what kind of a fist he will make of independent research. In his case, the dilemma arises prejudging who should be allowed to proceed from a Master's Degree to a Ph.D., as with a Ph.D. (at least in many countries) the person is overtrained for many industrial or teaching posts. The M.D. may well have no research experience during his six undergraduate and two hospital internship years. His decision to try his hand at research for the first time may thus come at age 26. If he invests two to three profitless years in finding out that he is not good at research, he ends up in a difficult situation.

I have said above that examination grades are the best available guides out of an unsatisfactory lot. Referee's reports, that is, confidential assessments by teachers who have known the candidate as an undergraduate, tend to be helpful if *negative* but not of much predictive value if eulogistic, as they usually are. Interviews may reveal personality traits that could cause clashes with a supervisor, but again many of the people gifted for research are somewhat queer fish, and a diffident or unusual interview presentation should not count against a candidate. A few beginners can be put off the idea of research when its real nature is revealed to them at interview, but frankly I have found interviews to be of far less help in judging scientific staff than for technical or ancillary staff. All of this adds up to the fact that, with the best will in the world, only perhaps one person in three that is picked to enter a programme designed to fit him for an academic post will in fact turn out to have sufficient research ability to make an effective medical academic in the present sense of the word. We must now ask, is such a system really wasteful?

Academics are often accused of empire-building when they take on more graduate students or untrained post-doctoral fellows than can find academic employment on the completion of their fellowship. Some selfish individuals really are guilty in this regard, treating the candidate as little more than slave labour. In most cases, however, the real reason is that only two years of exposure to bench science can sort the sheep from the goats. In most respects, the research training is not really wasted. The 'failed' research trainee is still a person of above-average ability. He should be able to choose and fill a responsible position in the community, and his exposure to the rigorous mental discipline of research should be of benefit in many fields. I have known 'failed' medical academics to tell me that those two or three years spent in research were amongst the happiest in their lives.

Nevertheless, it would be foolish to pretend that our relatively poor ability to predict who will succeed in research does not create big problems. There will be many people good enough to get a Ph.D. but not good enough to get a University job. In many cases, the realization of this comes as a shock to the individual. If medically qualified, he has a good way out in that he can go into specialist or general medical practise. If a science graduate, he must look to industry, government or some form of teaching at a level lower than the University. In many cases, employers in these categories are loth to take the Ph.D., feeling he may be overtrained for the job and unwilling to obey orders or stick to the task at hand. I feel that this represents a short-sighted policy. In most cases, the man able to go on and get his Ph.D. will be better than the one who stopped with a Bachelor's degree; he may in fact *make* the job that he fills into a more interesting and responsible one. At the present time, an over-supply of Ph.D's is a grave problem in many countries, and the whole issue needs careful study. However, any national policy about postgraduate training must take note of the fact that Universities can only be staffed by people who have filtered successfully through the advanced training described, and this will never reach one hundred per cent of the number who enter.

## Motivation of scientists

We have now seen a little of the qualities that go into making a research man, and have crossed a few of the hurdles that face him in reaching an academic post. What motives now lead the medical scientist on? Many of these are predictable. Being an intelligent and highly-trained person, he enjoys the challenge of a problem to be solved. The day-to-day manipulation of sophisticated equipment and the use of elegant techniques can bring the same kind of intense satisfaction that the artisan receives from his work well-performed. The wrestling with raw data needed to mould it into an understandable pattern; the planning of refinements in tomorrow's experiment based on today's results; and the gradual satisfaction of curiosity all bring joy and excitement. The final contemplation of a created work when a paper is at last published can give great pleasure. In other words, most successful scientists like what they do in a simple, intrinsic way.

The humanitarian aspect can also be a powerful motivating force in directing a young person towards medical research. I have known people to turn from physics, engineering or some other basic science to medical research chiefly for this reason. It is also heartening to see how readily most established scientists respond to specific appeals for the exercise of their talents in some humanitarian framework. For example, teaching programmes sponsored by the World Health Organization in Africa or Asia, even when involving weeks or months of work, are usually based around researchers drawn from all over the world. It is quite unusual for a scientist to refuse to be drafted on to an international committee or study panel convened to benefit or enlighten some public cause. In other words, scientists do not lose their desire to help mankind even after youthful illusions of great disease-shattering discoveries give way to a more mature assessment of individual limitations.

So far, none of these motives will cause surprise. We must now consider in some depth a source for motivation that is of very great importance but much less easy to explain to the lay reader.

### Peer-group recognition – A self-perpetuating goal in science

Sir Macfarlane Burnet has written that 'recognition of achievement is as important and necessary to the individual as food, shelter, security and affection'. Our age has perhaps cheapened the concepts of image and status, but the fact remains that for urban western man, the search for recognition and acceptance is a central driving force. In many walks of life, the degree of success achieved is measured with relative ease. For the industrial magnate, the size of his fortune and the empire he controls can readily be figured. For the executive, the importance of his firm, and of his position in it, will determine both salary and status. For the artist or musician, the size and faithfulness of his clientele or his audiences are easily assessed. As we move into professions like clinical medicine or the law, the lines become a bit more blurred. Indeed, the size of a practice and the esteem in which a man is held by his patients or his clients are readily evident, but the degree of respect which he commands among his professional colleagues will often be independent of this, and an important component of goal achievement. This is not to imply for a moment that businessmen are insensitive to peer group evaluation, but that the mensuration in objective terms of individual importance and worth is easier in their case. When we get to science, the peer group judgement becomes all-important. Except for the very occasional scientist who makes a discovery or invention either of world-wide immediate importance, or of direct applicability to some human problem, the objective measurement of individual contribution is quite difficult.

There are measures of scientific output, of course, but many of them are faulty. Probably the most widely-used single measure is number of scientific publications. On the other hand, one really good paper every two or three years is worth more than five 'pot-boilers' per year, so a quality-measure of some sort must be introduced. Here, the repute of the scientific journals in which a worker's papers appear is an important point. Some journals consistently publish only leading work in a field; others have much lower standards; and this comes to be widely known in the scientific community. Another measure which can be applied is to see how often a person's work is cited by other scientists. Papers of importance will serve as starting-points for further research, and will thus be quoted in the reference lists of other papers. An American publication, Science Citation Index, is compiled quarterly by computer and shows exactly where and how often a given paper is cited by others. This is a useful measure of the impact of work on the scientific community, but it also suffers from defects. For example, twenty authors may all cite a particular article saying it is *wrong*, and there is nothing to differentiate this from twenty citations all praising or confirming a piece of research. This is not as serious a limitation as it appears to be, because really bad papers are usually ignored by other researchers, and are thus rarely cited. Another limitation is that the number of citations will depend greatly on fashions; profound and important work going on in a field that is currently not very fashionable may be cited less frequently than its inherent worth merits.

Other semi-objective measurements of research ability that are available include the seniority of a person's position in his research establishment, the amount of financial support he can raise for his grants, the number of invitations which he receives to prominent congresses and symposia, the number and nature of scientific bodies with which he is affiliated, and so forth. In all of these, we already see subjective peer-group evaluation as a major contributory factor. As regards the progress of a young worker's career in the material sense, there is a very active 'old boy network' which is of paramount importance in advancement. If a young man is exceptionally able, this becomes known 'on the grapevine' with surprising speed, and he is inundated with job offers. If he is good but not exceptional, his supervisor's connections will be vital in placing him. We will examine this aspect more closely in Chapter 5.

We are thus in a position to state quite categorically that the chief factor both conferring and indicating a research worker's status is peer group evaluation. By this I mean an amorphous, unwritten but nonetheless real corporate assessment that scholars competent in a field reach concerning the ability of a given scientist. This concept is so important that it will dominate most of the rest of this chapter. Few scientists would deny the proposition that a desire to impress, gain the respect of, amaze with one's brilliance, or even prove wrong, a group of established scientists in one's sub-specialty is a real aspiration providing motivation and ranking prominently beside the motives already discussed. Indeed, a little reflection will show that desire for peer-group recognition is not unique to scientists. An actor wishes to be acclaimed as great by other actors; a writer will be as much pleased by praise from other literary figures as he will by a large royalty cheque. However, there is a difference for the researcher, as, perhaps more than any other creative person, he works in a field where the real nature of his achievement is upsettingly obscure to the common man. How *can* one explain at a cocktail party that the DNA-synthetic rate of a thymus lymphocyte is a vital issue that one has been wrestling with for months? It is much easier not to begin, allowing the questioner to dismiss you as 'another one of those inarticulate scientists'. Alternatively, one can sketch the broad outlines of a field, saying that one is studying the importance of immune defences in the cancer process, thus capturing audience interest; but this begs the question of an *individual's* worth, as perhaps one thousand scientists all over the world could, in all honesty, make this same broad statement. Communication with the layman is difficult, and recognition of worth by him dependent on indirect and often misleading cues. Therefore the part of a scientist's nature that wants and needs recognition increasingly looks inwards rather than outwards – towards the peer group rather than the general community.

This relative isolation of the scientist is a great pity. From his point of view it can easily lead to a pattern of living and thinking where his whole frame of reference becomes restricted to one small and atypical fragment of mankind. I know many scientists who draw virtually all their friends and acquaintances from amongst other scientists and who find it hard to take seriously the views and aspirations of 'ordinary' people. From society's point of view, the inward-looking tendency of research can breed disdain and disillusionment. The citizen slowly tires of seeing his tax dollar going on research that no one bothers to explain to him and that seems, at times, to advance with snail-like pace. There is room for a much more honest striving for communication from both sides of the fence, but the scientist particularly should re-appraise his position. In general, scientists who strive for some kind of recognition by, and identification with, the general community, through writing newspaper columns, appearing on popular science television or radio programmes and so forth, are looked at askance by their colleagues. Frequently they are dismissed as publicity-seekers or superficial blow-hards. Yet surely if more scientists sought to bring their work before a wider audience, albeit in simplified terms, both society and the scientist would benefit.

So far I have been intentionally vague in defining and characterizing these scientific peer groups. We must now examine their structure in more detail.

## The 'invisible colleges' and their influence

Professor Derek J. de Solla Price has coined the imaginative term of 'invisible colleges' to describe the international groups which set the fashions in modern science and constitute the chief peer groups to membership of which young scientists aspire. What are these invisible colleges? In a sense, they are clubs, but without rules or even strict membership lists. We have seen already that science is arbitrarily divided into major subjects, and that each of these may comprise twenty or more distinct sub-specialties. In each of these sub-specialties there will be active research, and by general consensus some of this will be more exciting and distinguished than the rest. In other words, there will be an international body of research workers, numbering perhaps fifty to a hundred people for each research area, who lead the world in that sub-specialty. These people will meet at frequent intervals, perhaps once a year or so, at some international congress or symposium. They correspond extensively among one another and exchange preprints and reprints. They visit one another's laboratories and exchange graduate students or post-doctoral fellows. They sit on editorial boards of specialist journals, and on committees recommending the allocation of grant funds. Occasionally they arrange complex international experiments with several different groups contributing a specialized technique towards the solution of a single problem. While the club has no corporate existence, and while at the outer limits it may be difficult to judge membership, its influence is very real and the 'hard core' of leaders relatively easy to define. Just as in the case of properly-constituted clubs there will be cases of overlap, with a given scientist identifying himself with two or three invisible colleges, distinct but with overlapping memberships. By the very nature of bench research, however, no scientist can belong to a large number of invisible colleges. The intense specialization of the invisible college differentiates it from other elements in the scientific power structure such as the Academies, the Government advisory panels and so forth. In truth, the colleges are very democratic – 'membership' is very readily extended to any scientist who makes a truly worthwhile contribution. In many respects, the up and coming under-thirty year-old with a recent, bright discovery is the most welcome member of a symposium sponsored by the club. Most scientists outside the magic circle think it must be very exclusive, while in reality the only entry qualification is some capacity to enrich the professional lives of the established members.

While the invisible college is a necessary and valuable part of the scientific scene, it is not without its disadvantages. We have already asked whether aspiration to membership might not contribute *too* greatly to a young scientist's motivation, to the exclusion of his participation in other human affairs. It is also true that invisible colleges are so attractive as to make voluntary abandonment difficult, and there is thus a certain self-perpetuating quality about sub-specialist groups that might continue to exist, have their symposia and so forth, long after the key research problems have been solved and any real need for that particular college has disappeared. Another thing that happens is that scientists of lesser gifts, unable to penetrate a college, seek to create a new one with most of the trappings but lacking real intellectual substance. Too often they succeed, and a kind of second-raters' club appears, leading to cluttering-up of the international literature with poor symposia or journals.

## Peer groups of more restricted influence

The definition of the invisible college is too imprecise for me to approach their description in strict numerical terms but as a first approximation one might guess that there are one hundred colleges for the biosciences, and ten thousand living scientists belonging to them. As there are at least one hundred thousand qualified graduates engaged in biological research the world over, it will at once be evident that many scientists never reach a college. It is my belief that for these individuals the general need to gain recognition amongst peers also applies. There are indeed collegial specialist groups with which good but less distinguished scientists can identify.

Chief among these are the local or national scientific societies, which exist for most major disciplines in most countries and even in many states or cities. These societies hold meetings, publish proceedings or abstracts and perform in their more restricted framework the same general functions as do the invisible colleges. Other peer groups will differ little from those existing in almost any organization. Obviously in Universities there will be graduate student associations; in an institute, little cliques will appear as circumstances dictate. The common feature for scientists in their interaction with any of these groups is that no need for justification or explanation of the general framework of activity exists. It is clear to the peer group that scientific research is a 'good thing', and interactions are on that basis.

**Peer groups of higher order and transcending sub-specialty barriers**

While the invisible colleges are probably the most important peer groups as regards the day-to-day conduct of research, there are certainly a good number of scientists whose place in one or more is so secure that higher goals are sought. Peer groups exist that transcend specialty barriers, and membership of which confers great status. Perhaps the best known of these is the Royal Society of London. Fellowship of this British institution makes one an 'F.R.S.', and C. P. Snow in his novels has written amusingly but accurately about just how important it can be for a research man to get into 'the Royal'. Many countries have an equivalent body; the U.S. National Academy of Science is an even more exclusive club, having a somewhat larger total number of members, but drawn from a much larger pool of career scientists. The most exclusive peer group of all is that of the Nobel Laureates. It is frequently stated that the achievement of a Nobel Prize is the ultimate goal for any scientist. I believe this statement to be an oversimplification. Many scientists will set their ultimate goal much lower, resting quite content with membership of an invisible college. Unquestionably some Nobel Laureates strive even higher, concerned perhaps with their ultimate place in history. There is a multi-layered hierarchical structure of peer groups, and a great degree of self-selection of goals, depending on a combination of ability, opportunity and degree of innate ambition. The key concept to recognize is the importance for scientists of esteem at the chosen layer.

For the clinical medical researcher, there is no real equivalent to the national academies, membership of which is traditionally confined to pure scientists. The Royal Colleges in England and Commonwealth countries, or the various national specialist boards in the United

States have much less exclusive membership policies, and operationally adherence to them is essential for practice of a specialty but does not confer great status. These bodies do excellent work, and constitute peer groups of practical importance, yet many authorities feel the desirability of some higher status outlet, such as national academies of medicine, for clinical scientists.

## Internationalism in science

We have said much in this chapter on the more selfish aspects of a scientist's motivation. It would be inappropriate to end this chapter on a negative note, as I truly believe scientists are neither more nor less selfish than any other group of intelligent, creative people. The most heartening thing about a lifetime in science, and an aspect that all researchers instantly recognize, is the international quality of research. In a world torn by tensions and prejudices, the realization by scientists that the quest for truth knows no national boundaries, that colleagues from obscure or even hostile nations can illuminate or transform one's work, is of immense practical and symbolic significance. In practical terms, one sees effects such as UNESCO, CERN, EMBO, IARC and the other supra-national efforts already discussed, international treaties governing space exploration, the international biological programme (IBP), the Pugwash movement and a myriad other attempts at collaboration. The symbolic element is even more important. The further a scientist goes, the more he realizes the widespread geographical nature of human intelligence; the more he matures, the more he values the achievements of his international competitors. Names on papers become faces at meetings, and before long, friends. The diversity in personalities and life-styles exhibited by scientists of different nationalities become such sources of enrichment of one's personal life as to transform its very nature. Prejudices give way to tolerance, soundly based on respect and affection. While only a proportion of scientists travel extensively, their friends, colleagues, students and other contacts share vicariously in the mellowing process. In many areas of research, scientists have learnt to live in *one world*. Is it too much to hope that their success will inspire other segments of mankind to do the same?

*Further reading*

P. B. Medawar, *Induction and Intuition in Scientific Thought*. Methuen, London (1969).

S. Ramón y Cajal, *Precepts and Counsels on Scientific Investigation and Stimulants of the Spirit*. Pacific Press, Mountain View, California (1951).
J. D. Watson, *The Double Helix*. Atheneum, New York (1968).

# 5

# The medical scientist – A pilgrim's progress

'*Both the man of science and the man of art live always at the edge of mystery, surrounded by it; both always, as the measure of their creation, have had to do with the harmonization of what is new with what is familiar, with the balance between novelty and synthesis, with the struggle to make partial order in total chaos*'.
R. Oppenheimer

Many gifted young people are attracted by the glamour attached to medical research but have little actual knowledge of either the nature of eventual career outlets or the steps leading up the ladder. A key aim of this book is to clarify this gradual pilgrim's progress for those readers either personally contemplating a research career, or bearing responsibilities for others contemplating this possibility. In this somewhat prosaic chapter, I will trace a student's progress from high school to final job, examining the changing nature of his contribution to research over the years. The aim is to sketch out the path from aspiration to achievement. It must be admitted that many find this path thorny, and wending its way through patches of boredom. Yet, in a very real sense, the above quotation from Robert Oppenheimer describes the real truth, and underscores the challenges and triumphs of a research career. May it serve as a beacon for those who find their spirits flagging during the early, passive stages of the learning process!

## Progress towards the Ph.D degree

While all the three worlds constituting the institutional framework of medical science, described in Chapter 3, employ both Ph.D. and medical graduates, in some cases in rather similar positions, there is a sufficiently great difference in career progression, particularly in the earlier stages, to warrant separate descriptions. Let us consider first the science student. Under the British and Australian systems, most science students leave the

University after three to four years' study with a bachelor's degree (B.Sc.). This qualifies them for a wide panoply of jobs, but in the Universities and research institutes that we are considering, a bachelor's degree suffices only for relatively lowly positions, mainly of a technical nature. After five years' study, a person is eligible for a Master of Science degree, which once was a prominent degree but now is regarded by most as a way-station to a Doctor of Philosophy (Ph.D.) degree. Operationally, therefore, most people completing a B.Sc. must then take a decision whether to go on to become a 'graduate student' for a Ph.D. In the United States, this involves going to 'graduate school'; after a fairly general education of four years in 'college', the student decides between a variety of graduate school possibilities which will include medical school or Ph.D. enrolment. For most young Americans, this also involves a change in institution and residence – it is relatively unusual to go to graduate school in the same college or university in which one obtained the bachelor's degree. The British and Australian systems are different. Here, there is no real equivalent to the traditional liberal arts college. Students leaving high school must opt then and there between medicine, science, dentistry, etc. For the science student, enrolment as a graduate student for a Ph.D. usually means staying on to do further study and research at the same university, though this is gradually changing.

What encourages some students to press on beyond the B.Sc.? The biggest single factor will be examination results or 'grades'. People with consistently high marks will usually be given preference for the scholarships and grants available, and will naturally regard themselves as best fitted to receive further education. A relatively small proportion of entering students will have had their minds on a research career from the outset, and these will most probably proceed to the Ph.D. unless poor results positively preclude them from so doing. In many cases, an individual professor can have a great influence on a person's choice. The student may meet a professor whose work or personality appeal to him, and if this teacher urges a research career, an important seed is sown. Much will also depend on the general home background and the moral support a student gets for such prolonged study. In most countries, the financial hardship involved in still being a student between the ages of twenty-two and twenty-six is eased by the provision of government-granted remuneration, which provides a modest living wage for a big proportion of the total number of Ph.D. students.

The nature of a Ph.D. student's work is radically different from that of an undergraduate. The number of set lectures and formal discussions or seminars goes down, and in the laboratory the candidate stops doing routine exercises and starts some research. Initially, this is under the direct supervision of one university man, and this first guide may be of crucial importance in determining a person's whole research life. The student, on the basis of his undergraduate likes and dislikes, makes a primary choice of major subject – biochemistry, physiology, microbiology and so forth – but his knowledge is rarely deep enough to make a considered choice of sub-specialty or detailed research area. Thus by a combination of personality assessment, consultation with the department chairman, and random forces of opportunity or chance, the student chooses *a particular* biochemist, physiologist, etc. as his thesis supervisor. In most cases, this man will have an ongoing stream of research, divisible into segments, but restricted to a small range of problems and scientific techniques. Amazing as it may seem to the lay reader, the problem area so haphazardly entered into at such a young age may define what sort of research a man may be doing fifty years later! Of course all sorts of changes in orientation will occur, but those early pre-doctoral years shape two things: peer group identification and technologic equipment. A student completing a Ph.D. thesis in virology *may* apply to do post-doctoral study in neurophysiology, but statistically is most unlikely to do so, for a variety of reasons. First, his familiarity with virology will leave him with impressions of a hundred experiments which he could continue straight away. Secondly, the techniques he has learnt would not be much good in a neurophysiology laboratory and he would have to start again from scratch. Thirdly, he may not know many or any neurophysiologists, but will have become acquainted with virologists both personally and through the literature. Fourthly, most neurophysiologists would prefer to take post-doctorals trained in their own discipline. None of these reasons may sound very good to the outsider, but they are solid, pragmatic ones with practical, everyday consequences. Few fresh science graduates realize all this when they enrol for a Ph.D. It never ceases to amaze me that they do not weigh more heavily the choice of their first supervisor in the light of the experiences of their seniors. The question ought to be one for study, reflection and research in its own right!

If the sub-specialty of one's first research supervisor matters, his intellectual quality and general research excellence is even more important. Should the supervisor be an internationally-known researcher, a member of an invisible college, he will impose high standards and judge performance sternly. If his protégé does well, the supervisor will help him to get into the big league. Opportunities for entry into another prominent laboratory for a post-doctoral study period will be facilitated. The post-doctoral period over, the candidate is ready for his first real job. Unquestionably his record of having come from two good laboratories will be a factor in his favour when the selection committee meets. In contrast is the situation where the young graduate chooses a nonentity for his first supervisor. Given ability equal to that of our previous example, he faces a much tougher battle. The mediocre man will impose less stringent standards, espouse lesser goals, give less enlightened supervision and certainly will have fewer contacts in first-rate laboratories to help in placing the candidate for post-doctoral study. Thus the second laboratory visited by the candidate may well be mediocre also. The man, on the average, will face his first academic appointments committee with a less impressive publication record and general background. I do not wish to imply that an outstanding person could not over-ride poor early experiences, nor am I completely happy about the system, some aspects of which have a nepotistic flavour. However, what I have described is a realistic assessment of the statistically likely results of this initial step, often so lightly taken. One sad part about this is that the student, whose whole future is at stake, often is not fully aware of the longer-range implications of his first choice.

Having considered the individual thesis supervisor, we should not forget the importance of the general academic climate which surrounds him. Early research experience is not a one to one relationship between supervisor and student. There will be other graduate students in the same and allied departments, other professors and lecturers involved in the same broad line of research, and in most instances the graduate student is part of a team. Obviously the quality of this larger universe will be as important in his formation as the quality of the thesis supervisor. There is a distinct tendency in research for gifted people to cluster around each other, so it will be unusual for the poor supervisor to be surrounded by brilliant colleagues or students, but on the rare occasion that this happens, it can be a student's salvation.

There is great difference of opinion on the question of how much independence graduate students should have in their work. At one extreme we have professors who do little more than outline a research problem and then leave the student to battle it out. Some men may have as many as a dozen Ph.D. students, frequently working on almost unrelated problems. In my experience, this system rarely works well. The student inevitably makes mistakes and much time may elapse before these are picked up. A programme run in this way can become fragmented and directionless. At the other extreme, we see quite a few research leaders who give their Ph.D. students such detailed directions that they become little more than intelligent technicians. This sort of programme can work well, both master and student getting more out of it than in the former case. However, I believe the best system lies between these two. The graduate student should get a project which is in the mainstream of the laboratory's research but sufficiently discrete to allow the student some personal identification. Initially, he needs close supervision but as his experience and confidence mount, this can be relaxed. There will clearly be much individual variation in the pace of increasing independence, but it is vital that there be a continuing two-way reaction, with the head of the laboratory reserving much time to listen to his student's ideas and plans. In fact, the young man with a fresh approach can make a big impact on the pattern of a laboratory's research, and there are few things more unfair than the lecturer who has no time for discussions with his research students, though unfortunately this is seen all too frequently.

At the conclusion of three to four years research, that is seven to eight years after entering university, the graduate student is ready to obtain his degree. In this period, he will have had a decreasing number of lectures and set education, an increasing involvement in original research. He may have a small number of papers in scientific journals, but the chief factor governing whether he gets his degree or not is a written document called a thesis. This consists of an analysis of previous research done in the field, in which the student sums up the status of knowledge and gives his ideas as to how the outstanding problems might be tackled. This section, called a literature review, is followed by the detailed presentation of experimental techniques and research results. A thesis usually allows a fuller, more leisurely treatment of all the minor facets of a piece of work than does a published paper. It can thus be a useful repository of highly technical information, and is kept on file in the university's library for future reference. Typically, a thesis would consist of a hundred and fifty to three hundred typewritten pages. The thesis is examined, usually by three scientists deemed to be competent in the field, one of whom is either the supervisor or another staff member within the sponsoring department, but two of whom are outsiders from other institutions or even other countries. Frequently, the student is given an oral examination as well, termed a 'defence' of the thesis, which can be quite a gruelling experience. For example, in France there is a tradition that this little ritual must expose the student to some of the best academic minds available and must severely test his mettle. Nonetheless, the thesis is the chief thing, and as few supervisors allow their students to hand in a sloppy thesis, it is quite unusual for a candidate actually to fail. What is far more common is that the student fails to make adequate progress in his research, and that it gradually dawns on him that he will never achieve enough for a thesis. In that case, the student may abandon his studies, settling for a Master's degree and some non-academic post.

## The post-doctoral fellowship period

In many countries, a useful interim period now begins, constituting an interlude between the end of formal education and the start of full academic employment in a university or institute. This is the post-doctoral fellowship period of two to three years. It has been recognized that experience in a laboratory remote from the by now familiar confines of the degree-granting university can be very broadening. For many this involves going to another country or even continent, and constitutes the first personal taste of the internationalism which is such a central part of academic life. Post-doctoral fellowships pay much better than undergraduate scholarships. For example, a typical stipend in the United States might be \$7000 to \$10,000 per annum. The post-doctoral system is most firmly entrenched in the United States and Canada, with governments paying the lion's share of the costs, and it is becoming increasingly important in countries like Britain, Australia and Germany. Unfortunately, it is much less established in some countries like France, Italy and Japan, where traditions in research have tended to be inward-looking and regressive. To the layman, the post-doctoral system may seem like feather-bedding. If a man has already been training himself for eight years, isn't it about time he did something useful for the community, such as teach practical classes? The fact is that the post-doctoral period may be the most productive time in a person's life. He is fully trained, yet free of non-research responsibilities. He has all the drive resulting from youth and the need to succeed. He has the great stimulation of a new environment to be appreciated and conquered. He is not yet bowed down with teaching, grantsmanship and administration. He is independent yet has a respected supervisor to give broad guidance. Little wonder that a significant fraction of the world's research is done by this admittedly privileged yet very positive force in academic life! The actual work done in the post-doctoral phase can be seen in terms of a natural progression from the Ph.D. period, and many of the variations in pattern described for the latter also apply to the former. There are two chief differences. First, it is universally accepted that the post-doctoral fellow has greater independence and carries greater research responsibility. Secondly, as the post-doctoral does not write a thesis, emphasis shifts to the need for the production of several sound scientific papers. The work published during the post-doctoral phase is one of the important visiting cards that the candidate takes to the committee interviewing him for his first job.

## The medical undergraduate and research training

Before we look at career progression in science any further, we must turn to the early research experiences of the medical student. In the British system, a course taking six years from high school leads to the medical degree, called 'M.B., B.S.' or Bachelor of Medicine and Bachelor of Surgery, the term M.D. being reserved for a higher qualification demonstrating expertise in research or some medical specialty. This is confusing to the layman as in the United States 'M.D.' signifies quite simply Doctor of Medicine, the degree received after four years in College and four years in medical school. In any event, both types of graduate are called 'Doctor' – strictly speaking a courtesy title in the British system as the graduate has no doctoral degree – and both must spend a year or two as junior residents (interns, housemen) in a major hospital before being able to practice medicine in the ordinary way.

The science student progressing to the Ph.D. spends a big proportion of his undergraduate life in a laboratory. The medical undergraduate, though taking part in some set laboratory classes, has, as the operational equivalent of the Ph.D's laboratory, the hospital ward. He must learn to interrogate, examine, diagnose, treat and also succour sick people. For the great majority of students, this is more appealing and glamorous than laboratory work. In short, for most the lab. represents an uninteresting chore that must be dispensed with as quickly and painlessly as possible. This leaves us, however, with a substantial minority of students, generally but not always the academically better ones, who have an interest in research. For these a variety of methods exists to allow them to learn their way around the laboratory a little better. Unquestionably it is the top American medical schools that have developed the most imaginative approach to encourage a research involvement in students. At medical schools like Stanford or Harvard, the annual intake of students is small and already highly selected. From their first year (which is, of course, their fifth year of tertiary education) students are encouraged to develop a liaison with one of their professors and to take part in a real research project in their spare time. During later years, many schools set aside an 'elective' period of several months during which students can work full time in research. Even in the lesser medical schools, students are encouraged to become familiar with the scientific techniques of the various diagnostic laboratories, and are given responsibilities for a limited number of these tests in the ward. In the traditional British system, classes tend to be bigger and real research possibilities for students more limited. One good alternative used by many universities is to allow a student to take off one full year for a research project during the middle of his course. He can, over that time, be regarded much like a Ph.D. graduate student, and can even qualify for an extra degree, such as the 'Bachelor of Medical Science'. Such a year can be of great inspirational value, and, in giving the student a glimpse of what the research life is really like, can allow him after graduation to contrast this with his hospital experience. Shorter 'electives' are also gradually gaining popularity.

It would be misleading to imply that all medical research means laboratory work. For example, a student may well find himself fascinated by a drug trial taking place in his hospital, or by a planned evaluation of some new surgical operation. This, too, is research. However, *most* clinical research endeavours have some laboratory component, even if it is only a laboratory analysis of blood or tissue from a large number of disease cases. Further, much clinical research rests in part on animal models of various sorts. In other words, it would be unusual for a person who actively disliked laboratory work to enter clinical research.

In many cases, therefore, the medical man finishes his course with less detailed knowledge of the research life than does the Ph.D. If academically inclined, he can now follow a number of different paths. He can take up a fellowship, usually after at least one hospital year, which may allow him to enter pure research and he may even take out a Ph.D., thus getting a double qualification. He may stay on the hospital resident staff for several years, developing a progressive interest in some specialty, and this may involve increasing exposure to clinical research. He may become a resident to a university professor which could lead to an invitation to join the junior staff of a university clinical department, where his responsibilities would include a mix of patient care, teaching and research. He may aspire to a senior position in laboratory hospital medicine, for example as pathologist or biochemist to the hospital. This can be achieved through senior residencies and various fellowships and junior positions; while these important posts involve mainly the routine application of existing knowledge, they do provide some opportunities for original research. Though the variety of paths to be chosen is greater, the general principles outlined for the Ph.D. still apply. In particular, the quality and renown of the young worker's sponsor plays an equally crucial role. Furthermore, it is becoming increasingly desirable for the medical graduate to have a postdoctoral experience away from his training institution. A variety of fellowship grant systems exists in the different countries to finance this. Therefore, in most cases, the young medical graduate approaches his first definitive job with two periods of supervised research behind him, much like the Ph.D. As the M.D. may well be several years older, and as other graduates from his age group in clinical practice will by then be earning high incomes, many academic institutions have had to introduce salary scales in which the M.D. receives considerably more than the Ph.D. for an essentially similar post. This is a continuing source of friction between the two professional groups.

## Graduates from faculties other than science and medicine

With the broad definition of medical research that we have adopted, we must consider also the role of other professional groups. Chief amongst these are graduates in veterinary medicine, dentistry, agricultural science and pharmacy. A veterinary surgeon can play a vital role in medical research. He may be in charge of the breeding, care and maintenance of experimental animals. He may study animal models of human disease. Also, he may make fundamental discoveries in basic science. A dental graduate may collaborate with a medical researcher in fields such as otorhinolaryngology, plastic surgery or microbiology. Agricultural scientists make prominent contributions in fields such as biochemistry and genetics. A graduate in pharmacy may go on and do useful work in pharmacology, the science of drug action. Graduates in any of these disciplines may go ahead and study for a Ph.D. and eventually may find employment in basic research, and the nature and scope of their work may be closely similar to that performed by medical or science graduates.

## Job outlets for research-oriented graduates

A complete listing of the job outlets for research-oriented M.D. and Ph.D. graduates is not possible here. Obviously, most graduates fit into one of the three worlds described in Chapter 3. There are, in addition, a few areas that we have not covered. In many cases, the large hospitals are inextricably wound up with universities, and the clinical research is done largely by university people. However, there are examples of where a hospital group is large and strong enough to sponsor a considerable amount of research while remaining outside the control of a university. Examples would include the Mayo Clinic, Cleveland Clinic or Kaiser Permanente Foundation in U.S.A. Also, many of England's great hospitals, though affiliated with universities, would loudly proclaim their own individual identity as separate institutions. In hospitals of this type, positions would exist with virtually full-time opportunities for research. As mentioned already, the vitally-important laboratory services of hospitals give their senior employees opportunity for research. In Chapter 3, I made brief reference to government-backed research institutes, and there are also public service posts where the appointee, though not formally a member of a full institute, is given some laboratory facilities for research. Indeed, there is a widespread recognition of the fact that in most scientific and technological fields, an employer will only obtain top quality brains if the appointee is allowed to make some kind of arrangement to perform original research.

Finally, we must consider briefly the unusual category of person who performs research in a commercial setting. There are individuals, small groups and even large institutions that contract, for a given fee, to investigate some problem on behalf of a paying client. This is more common in fields other than biology and medicine, and frequently involves highly specialized applied subjects that are perhaps more accurately described as development rather than research. Nevertheless, a 'knowledge industry' obeying all the normal commercial rules is emerging, and may well one day constitute an important segment of medical research.

For the rest of this chapter, we shall consider the university man and the research institute careerist as typical examples, hoping that the triumphs and trials of career progression will mirror those of researchers in other kinds of employment as well.

## The promotional ladder in academe

In universities, there is a reasonably rigid sequence of promotional steps dictated by a combination of age, length of service and accomplishment. Let us deal first with posts involving lesser responsibility and occupied by staff with limited ambitions. These can be in either teaching or research, and involve continued performance of relatively routine functions. Titles for such jobs include research assistant, research associate, demonstrator, senior demonstrator, etc. Rightly or wrongly, the occupant is frequently a woman, and staff at this level can provide an invaluable backbone for an organization. Apart from these categories, there are four levels of academic appointment. In order of increasing seniority they are termed lecturer, senior lecturer, reader and professor in the British system; and instructor, assistant professor, associate professor and professor in the American system. The nomenclature is further confused by the fact that in America the generic name covering all these posts in ordinary lay language is professor, while in Britain this word is reserved for the top post only. In both systems, the second level up is regarded as the 'normal' stage reached through seniority alone. Promotion to either of the higher two levels requires that the person be distinguished in some way. For the sciences, this usually means distinction in research. In most institutions, promotion is decided not by one man but by a committee, which also frequently solicits advice from experts outside the institution. The actual day-to-day duties of lecturing, demonstrating and performing research do not differ markedly in nature between the lower three categories, other than in the obvious respect of the more senior posts bringing more responsibility. In departments where there is only one full professor, the bulk of administration falls on him and the time available for research, and frequently even for teaching, is severely curtailed. Accordingly, many larger departments now have systems of two, three or occasionally even more full professors, with one acting as administrative head or chairman. This allows the other professors more time for research, and represents one way in which a university can hold its best research men.

Some universities are beginning to regard distinction in teaching as a major criterion for promotion, and this is a step which I welcome. In the nineteenth century and before, great prestige could accrue to a man renowned solely as a teacher. While not denying the importance of research in universities, it appears to me that the balance has swung too far in its favour, and any mechanism by which excellence in teaching can be rewarded will help both the public image of a university and its effectiveness in its prime aim of professional training.

In medical research institutes, there is much more variation in organizational pattern. I know one famous institute in which there are no set categories of seniority at all. There is a director, and there are research workers, the latter being all equal on paper. In this case the question of salary is negotiated individually and remains a confidential matter. In some institutes, there is a pattern very similar to the university one, and salary scales may be rigidly fixed by a government authority and are a matter of public record. In many institutes, there is a vaguely pyramidal system but with much scope for *ad hoc* changes left in the hands of the director or of a small committee. Once again, distinction in research overrides administrative or other abilities as the chief criterion for career advancement.

In most of academe, there is a controversial principle called 'tenure'. The legal status of this is frequently not iron-clad, but in practice, tenure means that the academic will not be dismissed unless he shows gross incompetence or commits some major indiscretion or crime. In America, tenure is usually associated with posts of associate professor or equivalent; in the British system it tends to come already with a senior lectureship. The tenure system has advantages and disadvantages. In its favour, it can be said that the mind of the academic possessing tenure is freed from worry about his personal financial security, and can thus concentrate on creative activity with full energy and without too many short-range considerations. Against the system one can argue that it protects the lazy and the mildly incompetent to an undue extent. From most practical respects, the argument is somewhat pointless as dismissals of academics of sufficient seniority to be eligible for tenure are quite rare. Some universities have strict 'up or out' rules – after seven years, a man must either be promoted to a tenure post or asked to leave, and I have heard this system criticized on the basis of depriving universities of the valued services of extremely competent and diligent, but unambitious and undistinguished 'backbone' workers. The Australian National Health and Medical Research Council has devised a tenure system which strikes me as fair and perhaps embodies most of the advantages and few of the disadvantages of a full tenure system. People of senior lecturer status and above are appointed initially for a period of five years. After this, their appointment continues indefinitely but the person can be given two years notice. This gives a good degree of security, allows plenty of time for the person under notice to rearrange his life, and retains a sufficient element of doubt of continuity to act as a spur when necessary.

## Problems of science administration

We have mentioned already that as a scientist progresses in years and status, his time for research becomes increasingly eroded by administrative responsibilities. I do not believe that any organization has found a perfect solution to this problem. It is frequently argued that researchers should have more non-scientific administrators on their staffs, and this can help. However, many of the problems that come up require a judgement by an experienced scientist, and the more able the scientist, the more valuable his opinion. This applies to issues as diverse as selection of professors, establishment of new institutions, governmental policies with respect to grant priorities, research training programmes, arrangement of conferences and congresses, and a host of others. As well as this type of administration, the senior scientist also gives a great deal of technical and conceptual advice, both within his institution and outside it. This activity has elements of both administration and teaching, and contributes to research output but *not* to the scientist's *own* research. In the last analysis, each individual scientist must adopt his own approach to this, making his own series of compromises and adjustments. There is no doubt that for many scientists, administration and committee work represent an escape from research as creativity and drive diminish. Few would admit this, even to themselves. An occasional top scientist is (or pretends to be) so poor at administration that his colleagues shield him from it and protect his interests. In the main, however, a scientist's non-bench responsibilities do increase with his seniority, and daily life becomes a difficult shuffling of competing priorities between various activities, each in themselves worthwhile. I have already expressed the firm belief that if a scientist wishes to contribute personally to the advancement of knowledge he must, with rare exceptions, devote a proportion of his time to an involvement in bench science. The likelihood of a substantial contribution is small if the time commitment falls below one-third of a working year.

## The scientist's changing role with advancing maturity

The wording of the last paragraph was chosen carefully, because an involvement in bench science does not necessarily imply the personal completion of an experiment from A to Z. Today, the process of discovery is a complex one, with many people contributing in different ways. Let us examine the changing role of a scientist's part in discovery with increasing maturity. The young scientist enters a laboratory or clinic in which a certain technical expertise and conceptual framework already reside. This resident corporate wisdom is usually regarded as the 'property' of the senior investigators running the laboratory, but experienced technicians may also play a big role, as they can often perform the actual experimental manipulations better than the chief scientist. Usually the graduate student is given a problem to attack and is told in precise terms what equipment and techniques to use in order to solve it. However, while the initial idea for the project may have been the supervisor's, the talented graduate student soon gets ideas and results of his own, which may modify or even radically change the direction of the research. The post-doctoral fellow will be even more inclined to exert an intellectual influence on experimental design. As the work progresses, at least in most of the laboratories that I respect, there is a complex and continuing interaction between the junior scientists, performing the bulk of the actual experiments, and the senior scientists running the laboratory. In the end, it is quite difficult to know to whom the discovery actually belongs! The system works best when the head man gets his hands dirty in some part of the experimental work. He may, for example, routinely perform some portion of the experiment demanding extra skill or judgement. On the other hand, he may maintain a closeness to the work by conducting personally a like but independent investigation on some related problem. He may choose not to pick up a test tube at all, but to observe very closely every detailed step of the experiment, giving advice or even orders on a strict day-to-day basis. In my estimation, all of this counts as 'bench involvement', and each senior scientists must decide how much physical laboratory work best fits his life-style. What I do *not* consider a bench involvement is to outline a problem to a junior colleague, and then to discuss the results with him three months later. This is still science, and a most valuable thing for a research leader to do; but if he does this full-time, he runs a grave risk of becoming disoriented and unrealistic.

The question of ownership of a discovery is not a trivial one. In truth, the ownership is usually shared, but both the nature of relative contributions and the generosity which governs apportionment of credit vary widely from laboratory to laboratory. As processes of patenting are rarely involved in the sort of research we are discussing, the accepted evidence of ownership is the authorship of the definitive published paper describing the discovery. Perhaps the most clear-cut proof of the importance of teamwork in modern research is the fact that the great majority of scientific papers now have from two to six or even more co-authors. In cases of co-authorship, it is accepted that the order in whch the names appear reflects the extent of their relative contributions; if all contributed equally, then the order is alphabetical. One practise that is widely used, but of which I personally do not approve, is that the head of the unit puts his name at the end of every paper coming out, regardless of the extent of his personal involvement. This is risky, as some people run such large laboratories that they cannot possibly know every detail of every experiment. Co-authorship means that a worker takes scientific responsibility for the content of the article. How can a man do this if what he knows about the work is confined to an initial interview and an occasional glance at pieces of paper with experimental results on them? If all the head of the laboratory has done towards a project is to give broad collegial advice and stimulation, the situation is adequately covered by the author's acknowledging this help in a footnote. If, on the other hand, the head has played a decisive and detailed role in experimental design and interpretation helping to shape the nature of the work on a daily basis, it may be appropriate for him to be a co-author even when he has not taken part in actual experiments. This situation arises often in a laboratory, and my personal attitude when it arises is to confine my co-authorship to the *first* paper that the junior person concerned publishes. This helps to get his name known and establishes the affiliation. Even though the intellectual relationship may not change, I believe it to be in a young person's interest not to perpetuate this 'sleeping partner' type arrangement.

**Elder statesmen in science**

So far we have concentrated our attention mainly on scientists who wish to maintain an involvement in bench research. For some scientists, this desire wanes in later life, and is replaced by a different kind of interest. I have said in Chapter 4 that research involves the need for an exceptional amount of drive, and many people over fifty just do not want to continue in this particular struggle. The fortunate thing is that there is still much that such potential elder statesmen of science can do which gives full scope to their talents and experience. The range of possibilities for the gifted man is wide. It includes Vice-Chancellorships of Universities, editorships of scientific journals, presidencies of scientific societies, positions on government expert panels, administrative posts in hospitals or research institutes and many others. Writing or lecturing on broad, philosophical themes can be fulfilling. A direr problem confronts the man of lesser distinction. While he is young, many may want his help essentially as an intelligent pair of hands. When he is middle-aged, teaching can fill a gap, but in science it takes much energy to keep up with changing trends, and effectiveness in teaching diminishes rapidly if the drive to keep up with research knowledge recedes. Therefore, the ageing scientist of modest ability may find himself with nothing much to do, looking with envy and some fear at the army of young men coming along; they seem so much fuller of ideas. As in most aspects of life, the solution to this dilemma is to be found in self-knowledge. The man who appreciates these changes in himself as normal physiological processes can find dignity and fulfilment in lending his skills to the services of the creativity of others, but unfortunately it is rare in practice for an older scientist to follow this path. Indeed, academe has found no overall way out, and most departments simply carry a proportion of what is unsympathetically termed 'dead wood'. Society as a whole may soon have to face the general problem of how the skills and experience of older people can best be harnessed.

This analysis makes no pretence at completeness. In particular, its intentionally realistic tone has not allowed the mystery and the thrill involved in research to emerge. Maybe there is no need for me to state in so many words how fulfilling a research career can be. The very writing of this book is an expression of my faith!

*Further reading*

D. J. Ingle, *Principles of Research in Biology and Medicine*. J. B. Lippincott Co., Philadelphia, (1958).

D. C. Pelz and F. M. Andrews. *Scientists in Organizations. Productive Climates for Research and Development.* John Wiley and Sons, Inc. New York (1966).

H. Selye, *From Dream to Discovery: on being a Scientist.* McGraw-Hill, New York (1964).

# 6

# The role of government policy in medical research

'*Science, broadly considered, is incomparably the most successful enterprise human beings have ever engaged upon*'. P. B. Medawar

The second half of the twentieth century will probably be remembered as the period during which man's love affair with science passed the honeymoon phase. The previous hundred years had represented one of those rare surges of mankind's creativity, episodic, unpredictable, cosmic in its impact, which changes irrevocably the course of history. In that relatively short time, representing a little more than one percent of the span of civilized existence, science and technology had become the new power currencies of global politics. Around 1900, medical research found itself well in the mainstream of this historic tide. Pasteur, Lister, Ehrlich, Koch and their many colleagues had left a legacy of vast import; few could have challenged the view that the new creativity, based on science, was fashioning a braver future. By 1950, the discovery of vitamins, hormones, antibiotics and a host of other drugs and treatments had placed medicine on a scientific footing and no ill appeared unconquerable. Now, despite the fact that more people than ever before are using their minds to combat ignorance, we have lost our way. To a surprising extent, we are being carried along on a world-wide wave of pessimism about science and technology. The faith that man's creativity can be a cause for hope has been replaced by a despair which casts scientific research and technology as a kind of villain.

Yet, Sir Peter Medawar's claim quoted above is probably valid. The world-wide capitulation to science and technology, in fact for the developed world and in aspiration for the undeveloped nations, lends credence to his view. What went wrong? The physical sciences are most prominently involved, with the threat of nuclear annihilation holding centre stage. A current catch-cry, namely technology as the despoiler of the environment and quality of life, is fast challenging as the chief weapon of the critic of science. Medical research has not escaped from criticism. The horrors of biological warfare are evident, but equally powerful is the more subtle, slow realization that the therapeutic triumphs of the last fifteen years have not been as good as originally foreshadowed. As a result, there is a growing sense of disillusionment with medical research in some quarters. This is at least partly the fault of the medical research establishment itself, which justifies its many appeals for public funds by promises for advances in treatment frequently cast in less than judicious terms. In this chapter, we will examine the reactions of government to this changing pattern of community attitude to medical research.

## The extent of government financial involvement in medical research

In Chapter 3, we saw that government grants had become the main source of finance for medical research in universities and research institutes, be these governmental or private. In fact, medical research has become a substantial industry. Taking a broad definition and including also biological research, the 1974 national expenditure for medical research would be around $US 2,500,000,000 for U.S.A.: £40,000,000 for Great Britain; $A 15,000,000 for Australia. At least two-thirds of these overall costs are borne directly by governments. Interestingly, though these sums seem substantial in absolute terms, they are still only a small percentage of total national expenses on health. Of course, the lion's share of the money goes on health care delivery. In the United States, the 'medical-industrial complex' is still largely a private enterprise affair. Its total costs are estimated at around $US 75,000,000,000 or around seven per cent of the gross national product. About forty-two per cent of this huge bill is the cost of running hospitals and nursing homes; twenty-six per cent goes in payments to medical practitioners; another eleven per cent represents the cost of drugs; and viewed as a percentage, research expenditure comes out at a modest three per cent. This percentage is still much higher than that which pertains in other countries. Thus, the British National Health Scheme costs around £2,500,000,000 per year and total health expenditure in Australia is around $A 2,000,000,000. In other words, research expenditure in the two countries represents 1.6% and 0.75% of total health costs.

Two points emerge from this analysis. The first is that medical research expenditure is large and thus a proper concern of governments. The second is that it is small as a percentage of total health care costs. In fact, the research effort in any country could be doubled or trebled without any marked direct effect on total health expenditure. This second point is worth stressing, because in the United States today one hears the frequently-voiced feeling that the priorities have somehow become mixed up; that research has been pushed ahead at the expense of adequate health care delivery, and that the health of the nation has suffered as a result. There may be some truth in that claim if viewed in purely symbolic terms. Perhaps academics and professional leaders have laid unduly great emphasis on the value of research. However, in straight practical terms, the academic is 'small cheese' when considered in the total health framework. His extravagance in research, if indeed such did exist, could hardly affect the wider problem. The difficulties in health care delivery systems are of an altogether larger scale. It is a little unfair to make the academic a scapegoat for the larger and essentially political problems of the medical industrial complex.

## Current patterns of medical research financing

As the United States sets the pace in medical research financing, we can take this country as our first model of how government support really operates. We saw in Chapter 3 how governmental granting agencies took over progressively from private foundations as the sheet-anchor of most research programmes. Of central importance is a branch of the U.S. Department of Health, Education and Welfare known as the N.I.H. (National Institutes of Health). Under the directorship of Dr. James Shannon, N.I.H. expanded rapidly between 1950 and 1965, its budget rising to over $1,000,000,000. The majority of this sum was expended as extra-mural grants to aid research in institutes and universities. A remarkably effective peer-group evaluation system has been set up to administer the grants. Grant requests coming in from investigators are assigned to study sections made up of leading active investigators in some dozens of research fields. Emphasis in selecting members of study sections is placed on current research productivity and not on seniority alone. Moreover, study section membership is for a three to four year term only, and thus no single person holds power for very long. Each project receives as thorough and objective a review as possible, and is given a priority rating by the study section, based on an assessment of its scientific merit. A second administrative body, a council consisting of more senior scientists and administrators, reviews the study sections' decisions, and may make some minor adjustments based on an assessment of the relevance of projects to U.S. health goals. Until fairly recently, this function was rarely exercised by councils, which acted in the main as a rubber stamp for the study sections. In the last five years, councils have been rearranging priorities more extensively, and some acrimonious reactions from study sections have resulted. Nevertheless, the review system overall is considered a model of fairness by the actual consumer, the working scientists themselves. While N.I.H. takes a very broad view of the definition of health-oriented research, and supports basic as well as clinical research, there is a second government agency called N.S.F. (National Science Foundation) which gives grants for pure research projects in the biosciences. This operates on a system rather similar to that of N.I.H. Many scientists file duplicate grant requests to N.I.H. and N.S.F., and allow administrators to sort out which body will support their research. The chief virtue of the dual system is to ensure that if an investigator, for one reason or another, falls foul of one study section, he can have recourse to a totally independent review by a separate body.

In the United Kingdom, patterns of medical research financing will be greatly influenced by the Rothschild report. This, in effect, urged that medical academies should be more concerned with applied research, and that a bigger proportion of available research funds be expended on goal-oriented, defined projects, supported through contracts, rather than the traditional investigator-initiated and more open-ended research projects. It is proposed that some of the funds will flow through the Department of Health directly, rather than through the Medical Research Council (perhaps deemed to be a little too 'pure' in its orientation). In the face of a distinct plateauing of all research funds in the United Kingdom, the long-term impact of the proposals will be considerable.

We cannot here describe in detail the way in which other countries attack this problem. Suffice it to say that most have a dual system, with 'health-oriented' and 'pure science-oriented' granting bodies. As a general rule, few countries have a review system quite as expert and democratic as that in the United States, in part because of the smaller number of real experts available to serve on study sections. Moreover, no country has comparable sums to expend, even on a *per capita* basis. There seems, however, to be a trend right throughout the developed world to expend more on medical research and to follow the lead given by U.S.A.

## Recent trends in U.S. research financing

Even the most enthusiastic supporter of medical research could not have hoped for an indefinite growth in medical research effort at the rate characterizing the 1950–65 period. Unfortunately, however, a series of events over the period 1965–1974 conspired to make the fiscal scene for medical and scientific research in the U.S.A. very bleak in comparison to a decade perviously. As many countries tend to imitate U.S. trends some years later, we must examine these factors closely.

The first factor which has led to plateauing of U.S. government support for medical science is the fault of the scientists themselves. Buoyed up by some of the spectacular successes of the post-World War II years, and in particular by the dramatic development of effective vaccines against poliomyelitis, some leading scientists began to make extravagant claims for what medical research might do, given adequate funding. Prospects for cures for cancer and prevention of heart disease were widely proclaimed. Many investigators, engaged in projects that were ninety-five per cent pure science, were encouraged to publicize the possible relevance of their work to human disease, and especially to cancer. No serious attempt was made to sort out short-range goals, achievable by steady application of known principles, from long-range goals, including projects with a high risk factor. Any thoughtful scientist could have said in 1950 that the solution of polio (the cause of which was known) was an incomparably easier task than the solution of heart attacks (the cause of which was and is largely unknown). In fact, few researchers bothered to do so, and the voices of these few were drowned out by the many who simply wanted more money for research and gave no thought to an eventual day of reckoning.

A second factor leading to less funds for research was the realization by the U.S. Congress that research discoveries were being unevenly applied. Some U.S. citizens, those finding their way into the most high-powered, research-oriented clinics, got the most advanced medical care in the world. Many others were victims of failures in the health care delivery machinery, and had access to extremely sub-optimal care. This realization sparked off a series of programmes aimed to ensure wider spread and application of known discoveries throughout the medical community. President Lyndon B. Johnson started an ambitious 'cancer, heart disease and strokes' programme designed to foster earlier diagnosis and better treatment of these disorders. In the congressional mind, these projects came to take precedence over conventional research. The re-orientation has had one good effect. It has made university academics more conscious of the importance of communicating discoveries to practitioners, especially those not closely connected with centres of academic excellence. In the main, however, it was pointless to raise a contrast between research and health care delivery, as the latter is so much more expensive, and involves a host of administrative and social problems as well as scientific ones.

The third factor, leading to lessened research funds was a justifiable concern about quality control. At the time when it was government policy to push research very hard, almost anyone with a degree and a half-way respectable research idea could get a government grant. In the desire to get much research off the ground as quickly as possible, many investigators of mediocre quality were funded. While this may have been conscious policy, a certain multiplier effect may not have been considered sufficiently. These mediocre researchers in their turn produced graduate students, who eventually obtained their degrees and began clamouring for grants. For a while, the amount of funds for research increased fast enough to satisfy the available manpower pool. Around 1965, the pattern changed and research grants levelled off without warning. Academe did not react quickly in reducing graduate student intake, and moreover many people were in the midst of their training. It took till about 1970 for the full gravity of the situation to become clear, and graduate school enrolments are now down somewhat in the U.S. However, the young scientist finds himself in a difficult situation, not of his making, where he is competing with his seniors for limited funds. The strain is being felt particularly in pure scientific, non-clinical areas. In the long range, the current concentration on support of only excellent research programmes may have the beneficial effect of causing people of modest ability to find employment in fields more suited to their gifts, but in the short range, the 'stop-go tactics' have caused considerable dislocation and human distress. It further would be well to recall J. B. S. Haldane's dictum that 'pure science is science that hasn't yet been applied'. It is clear that research financing needs careful national long-range planning.

## World-wide trends in research financing

I have said that the world has trailed America in the financing of research by some years. This has led many top scientists to move from countries like Canada, Great Britain, Germany and Scandinavia to the United States, causing the famous phrase 'brain drain' to be coined. One apparent benefit of being an imitator is that, potentially at least, he can avoid mistakes and excesses. Thus most countries, with financial commitments much smaller as a proportion of GNP than those of the U.S., have been able to continue a steady, unspectacular build-up in medical research. An exception is Canada, which from 1967 on greatly accelerated its national effort and must strive hard not to repeat U.S. mistakes. Many countries, including Australia, are starting to reverse the brain drain and to develop granting patterns which, though less lavish than American ones, give promise of the eventual emergence of a stable, satisfactory system. We must now examine what the essential features of a good governmental policy in medical research should be.

## The importance of long-range planning in government science policy

The first and most integral part of any research programme is the scientific manpower. The amount and quality of medical research that can be performed in a country depends on the number and ability of its medical scientists more than on any other variable. The training of a medical scientist, as we have seen in Chapter 5, is long and expensive. Therefore the first desideratum of a national medical science policy is that reasonable projections are made about the numbers of medical academics that will be required in the future, and about the nature of the career outlets available to them. This is no easy exercise, as the number will depend on many factors other than simply the desire for research output. Amongst things requiring consideration will be the number of doctors a community wants, which in its turn dictates the number and size of medical schools required; the number of major hospitals and the size and nature of their scientific staffs; and the structural framework of non-university academic institutions. When it is clear how many medical scientists should be trained, it will be possible to determine the number of graduate student scholarships and post-doctoral fellowships that should be made available, programming in some reasonable factor of wastage. Attempts should be made at national level to co-ordinate the timing of training programmes with progressive availability of new jobs. I recognize that the necessary projections will contain inaccuracies, and that changing economic circumstances may alter the pace at which jobs become available. However, I believe that the probability of deficiencies in any plan is no excuse for having none at all. At present, in most countries, patterns of medical research financing represent a patch-work quilt of *ad hoc* decisions based largely on shifting power relationships of various pressure groups. I want to preserve some entrepreneurial aspects on a backbone of stable long-range government planning, thus hoping to combine the best of two worlds. In particular, long-range planning could avoid the worst disappointments inherent in sudden cut-backs, and could provide medical scientists with a basis for their own individual planning of careers and staff policies.

## Research costs as a percentage of health costs

An objective determination by a government as to how much it should spend on medical research is by no means easy. Presumably each country has a certain image of itself in terms of the degree of its development. Countries like the United States, Great Britain or Sweden have a history of being in the forefront of research. Most Asian, African and South American countries expend the bulk of their intellectual and financial effort not on research but on application of established knowledge to social problems. Many countries, for a variety of reasons, are in the intermediate position of having little past history in research but a desire to expand future activities. In each situation, a persuasive case can be made for relating the total national expenditure on medical research to total health costs. Any industrial corporation also faces the essentially arbitrary decision of just how much to spend on research, and in many cases, a guideline is taken from annual sales figures. The large pharmaceutical houses consistently set aside ten per cent of sales for research. No doubt the figure is much lower for other industries, and even higher for a few. In any country, the aim of expending money on health is no doubt to improve health. In the long run, new research discoveries are a basic component of this process of progressive improvement, and an investment in research is a long-range investment in world health. It therefore seems logical that a relationship should exist between research expenditure and the overall dollar commitment to health. When national efforts in medical research are viewed in this light, some surprising statistics emerge. For example, though realizing that Australia's per capita expenditure on medical research was low, I was quite surprised that the annual total came to less than the cost of a government scheme which provides a glass of free milk per day for all Australian school children! It further emerged that total medical research expenditure (governmental and private) was less than one-twentieth of the annual expenditure on drugs. It seems important that such statistics be collected in an orderly way and be the subject of political debate. I feel certain that many thinking people would express some surprise at the relatively low cost of research, and would have sympathy towards a plan that projected a gradually-rising expenditure reaching a target figure of some two to three percent of total national health costs.

### Medical research versus research in other fields

A sensible policy about health-oriented research must of necessity take into account the level of research in other fields. There are many spheres of human activity able to be benefited by research, and also there exist fascinating pure research problems in many fields that are unlikely to yield information of practical value. It is reasonable that some balance be maintained between the various research areas. There are some authorities who make a persuasive case against any overall national science policy, feeling that the ebb and flow of natural, impulsive forces will lead to a situation that society will accept. One of the strongest arguments against this viewpoint is the realization of the sorts of imbalances that can develop in national science expenditures. For example, A. M. Weinberg has presented statistics relating to U.S. national expenditures in the year 1965. The total Federal Government expenditure on research and development was $16,000 million. Of this, $8,000 million was spent on military research, $5,000 million on space research and over $1,000 million on health research. While admiring the fantastic feats of the space programme, I cannot help feeling that most voters would find the imbalance between the latter two figures somewhat curious. The U.S. President has a science advisor and a national science council, and one might hope that amongst their chief duties would be an arrangement of priorities and wise balancing of competing research demands. At the very least, each country should have an accurate governmental machinery for determining how much is being spent on different areas of research, so that any clear-cut anomalies can be recognized and corrected.

## Short-range versus long-range goals in medical research

I have already alluded to the fact that over-enthusiastic claims for immediate solution of disease problems by medical academics has led to Congressional disillusionment in the U.S. Over the immediate post World War II period, governments came to look on better clinical medicine as a regular and predictable outcome of adequate research financing, but medical science is much too complex and multifactorial an entity to obey any simple growth curve. Our power to prevent and treat disease will increase, but at a pace that will be irregular and unpredictable. The major breakthroughs will emerge, probably quite capriciously, in a climate where a solid base of pure science exists. Scientists must educate legislators and the public to a realistic acceptance of the difference between short-range and long-range research goals. Work on the ultrastructure of cells, the function of enzymes, the replication of nucleic acids, must be financed and justified in the context of long-range objectives. A continuing commitment to basic research must be regarded not as a bus stop on the route to a cancer cure (as it has been in the past), but rather as a necessary springboard for all subsequent progress in more applied areas. In a climate where these issues are fully appreciated, governments and their expert committees can then come to the essentially political decision of how much money to expend on the short-term, clearly applied goals versus the long-term ones. It would be my hope that at the end of this educational process, legislators in the more developed countries would allocate about half of the available funds to the long-range type of project. There may be a serious problem in communication here. Perhaps scientists underestimate the intelligence and goodwill of politicians, and politicians underestimate the sophistication of voters. In a world that is becoming increasingly educated, a franker, fuller discussion of the role of research might turn out to be good politics.

## The controversy over the usefulness of research

So far in this book I have tended to discuss medical research as a form of activity which is good and worthwhile because it may yield knowledge leading to an improvement in human well-being. There is a strong body of opinion, particularly amongst scientists themselves, that holds this type of justification to be neither accurate nor necessary. Proponents of this view point to the fact that a large part of the day-to-day impetus in a scientist's life is derived from a desire to know, a joy in the process of discovery. Thus knowledge is deemed to be valuable for its own sake quite apart from any impact which that knowledge might have on practical human affairs. The activities of the researcher are seen largely as exercises of the creative human spirit, comparable to those of an artist, writer or composer. Taken to its extreme, this viewpoint regards research largely as an immensely satisfying sort of game. Its chief usefulness to society is taken to be the fact that it employs people in work not producing consumer goods needing, in their turn, to be sold.

While I consider this attitude worthy of deep study, I am concerned to see it placed as an antithesis to the concept of usefulness of research. Rather, I see it as a description of an additional, complementary characteristic. Research is creative, is a highly amusing game *and* is at all times capable of yielding knowledge which affects man's future. Let us take as an example of pure research the field of astronomy applied to stars outside our galaxy. At first sight, this may seem an exercise incapable of yielding practical results. The stars observed may be millions of light-years away, may have ceased to exist, and any prospect of getting to them or communicating with them may be impossibly remote. Nevertheless, a closer look shows innumerable ways in which this type of research may be 'useful' in quite a conventional sense. It may yield information about the nature of light, or of space, or of radio waves, or of matter, vitally significant to earthly problems. Moreover, it is useful in the less obvious ways of enlarging man's understanding of the universe and of his restricted role in it. Search as one might for examples of research that are truly 'useless', the relatedness of all portions of the physical universe is such that no validly performed experiment can be confidently tipped as qualifying!

The attributes of pleasure and of potential usefulness of research are separable, of equal descriptive value, and non-competitive. Which one chooses to highlight or dissect will depend on the nature of the task at hand. When one discusses the place of research in modern society, as is the central aim of this book, it is fitting to consider both aspects. When one decides in a political setting what, and how much, research to do, it seems reasonable that more weight be given to the concept of usefulness. In neither case does it seem logical to create a contrast.

## Indirect escalation of medical care costs through research discoveries

Research itself, as we have seen, is a surprisingly minor expense item in a nation's health bill. However, research has contributed greatly to escalating health costs in a more indirect way. New and elaborate diagnostic techniques, expensive new drugs, a proliferating need for highly-trained paramedical personnel, need for multiple specialists to see difficult cases in consultation, are all in effect the results of the success of medical research. How should this fact affect a national medical research policy? In my opinion, three factors should dominate thinking here. First the spread of medical information throughout the developed world is now rapid and effective. If an advance of real practical value is made in one country, the lag time before pressure builds up in the medical communities of other countries for its local application is, at most, two to three years. It could, therefore, be argued that a reduction of expenditure on research by any one country will affect this indirect cost escalation relatively little, so long as other countries continue to do research at an undiminished pace. Of course, the argument can equally well be turned around and used, in smaller countries, as an excuse for *not* doing research, as the fruits can so readily be imported. We will have occasion to discuss this aspect in Chapter 7. From our present viewpoint, it would seem that the only nation which could, by unilateral decision, materially reduce world medical research output (thus reducing the indirect cost escalation) is the United States of America. As any large reduction there does not seem likely, the indirect cost factors should not affect other countries' medical research policy.

The second factor to consider is the economic saving of many major advances. For example, sanatoria for chronic tuberculosis and poliomyelitis after-care, both very expensive items, have virtually disappeared since research provided effective control of these diseases. Pressures on mental hospital facilities have eased. Less time is lost from work when illness is promptly treated. The one major economic problem created by medical research that is not yet being tackled effectively is that of increasing numbers of aged people.

The third factor relates to changing attitudes of more affluent communities towards consumer products. It is frequently stated that a community's capacity for absorbing more and more material goods is insatiable. I believe this to be untrue, or at least oversimplified. Many communities in affluent nations are beginning to clamour for less emphasis on material consumption and more on quality of life. Few things are as essential to enjoyment of life as good health. If this less materialistic wave of today's young thinking spreads, as I believe it will, so a desire for more medical research will become manifest. A good national science policy must attempt to assess the strength of such trends.

## Avoidance of extravagance in national science policy

We have already discussed the imprecisions in the assessment of scientific output and merit. An allied problem is the control of expenditure on given lines of research. Most expenditures of governments have clearly visible results – armies, hospitals, schools, roads. As most medical research discoveries are non-patentable, the results of an enlightened science policy have to be assessed on vague criteria such as prestige and the catalytic effects of excellence in research on other fields such as education, medical practice, and so forth. Furthermore, non-scientists, and thus governments, have no way of assessing what a scientist *really needs* to pursue his research. If an acknowledged expert in a scientific sub-specialty claims to need an instrument costing $30,000 as an essential item in his research budget, no bureaucrat can counter the claim. In other words, no outside control is possible – the only protection against extravagance must come from within science itself. It is one of the great responsibilities of the scientific community in any country to exert self-control in spending. Irresponsible attitudes could produce short-term advantages, but in the long run must produce political disillusionment. The detailed disposition of available government medical research funds must be under the control of the scientists themselves. A nation must work out a grant review system that is thorough, fair and reasonably tough. The experts on review panels must have enough technical knowledge to distinguish real leadership and enterprise from mere 'grantsmanship'. In the smaller countries, this is not as easy as it sounds. There are many scientific sub-specialties, and when large grant requests come from the most renowned leaders of any given one, there may not be many independent reviewers able (or willing!) to give the proposed projects objective scrutiny. In such cases, it may be wise to seek an assessment from a foreign group of experts.

While the most obvious potential source of extravagance may be the large, active research group, the most pernicious source comes from quite a different direction. It is through unnecessary patience with unproductive, poor quality research. Frequently one sees the budget of a really productive group cut by a committee and the funds thus made available dissipated on a number of smaller and totally mediocre projects. It is clearly very difficult to maintain an equitable balance between support of established leaders, and funds made available to younger, untried investigators or to groups starting off in new universities or institutes. I am all in favour of liberality in the latter two directions, but this must be accompanied by realistic deadlines. If, five years after getting his first grant, a scientist still has not produced any worthwhile research, his statistical chances of doing so in the following five years are small and his next grant assessment must be correspondingly tougher.

From the viewpoint of government policy, the need for peer group grant reviews is widely recognized, and the key decision in this area is whom to put onto the review committees. Here it is essential to achieve a good balance of active working scientists, leaders in their fields and *au fait* with current trends; and more senior scientists, slightly above the battle and possessed of extra experience. The former group should be in the decisive majority. The latter group have a very real role, too; but frequently, especially in European countries, their numbers and power are too large.

Another mistake that government committees frequently make is a failure to achieve a good balance between the four major categories of scientific expenditure, namely scientists' salaries, technicians' salaries, permanent equipment and consumable scientific supplies. It is not uncommon to see a request for a $40,000 electron microscope pass with little trouble, but a budget of $1000 for chemicals or glassware to be arbitrarily cut in half. Similarly, the need for expert technical assistance is frequently underestimated. These mistakes are least common when working scientists predominate on committees.

## Project versus institutional support of research

A difficult decision which each nation must make is how to divide the total available research budget into project support versus institutional support. By project support I mean funds that can be competed for by investigators from any institution, usually involving commitments of three to five years' duration, and assessed purely on the merits of the individual investigator and his project. Institutional support means the long-term underpinning of a staff establishment and other costs of research, regardless of short-term successes, staff changes or even changes in the direction of an institute's research. Each form of support has its advantages and disadvantages. Project support allows virtually continuous review of productivity, adjustment of national research goals, and rapid expansion of unusually promising lines of research. It does, however, tend to slant an investigator's research strategy towards short-range goals; the 'publish or perish' attitude is strengthened and grantsmanship skills may be unduly rewarded. The truly thoughtful researcher with some long-range, profound dream may suffer. Institutional support provides stability, allows long-range planning at the level of both investigator and institution, and saves the scientist from becoming too much of an entrepreneur. However, in the absence of talented leadership, the institute that is too stably supported may lose impetus. People become comfortable, the need to perform with continued excellence is less, the pace and ferment may become suboptimal. An ideal national system should encompass both types of support, and institutions that are totally financed by government institutional support should come under thorough independent review every five years, using the same stringent criteria of worth as are applied to project grants. Universities should receive a modest baseline of institutional research support, spread evenly amongst departments, and access to competitive project grant funds.

## Support of centres of excellence

A strong case can be made out for special treatment by review committees of certain centres that are exceptionally outstanding. In most countries, there are a very few groups that are universally identified as having created centres of excellence around them. As a general principle, money granted to such centres is a fool-proof investment, especially in regard to training of younger workers. Also, the time of such leaders is valuable and should not be unduly taken up with the paper-work of grantsmanship. As well as being a source of national pride, such centres can also create considerable jealousy amongst less gifted academics, and it is possible for standard review committees to be biased through this. Each specific instance may well require a different national policy, but a fiscally permissive attitude, subject again to periodic review, is the appropriate one in such cases.

## Subject areas for research in a country

One of the most controversial questions facing each nation is whether there should be some central direction deciding which areas of research work should be supported. In the United States, the scientific manpower and financial resources are such as to allow virtually all fields of medical research to be covered. This is not completely true for any other country, including affluent ones like West Germany or traditional leaders in science such as Great Britain. The problem is especially pressing for countries with a small population, such as Sweden, the Netherlands or Australia. For these nations to compete in an international framework, they must restrict their research horizons to encompass part only of the total spectrum of sub-specialties. If scientists form themselves into tight-knit groups in this way, a small nation can make a large impact. Thus, to choose a few examples, Sweden is strong in neurosurgery and biophysics; the Netherlands in radiation biology and pathology; Australia in neurophysiology and immunology. How does this come about? How do nations decide in a conscious way to expand this or that area of research?

Traditions, often dating back to some early key figure, are an important factor. France's concentration of effort in microbiology dates back to the school built up by Pasteur in the nineteenth century; Sweden's biophysical strength owes much to the work of Svedberg and Tiselius in the 1930s; Australia's emphasis on immunology rests very definitely on the seminal influence of Burnet. It makes good sense for a nation to capitalize fully on such traditions and to stake out an ongoing world reputation on them, as unquestionably excellence breeds excellence in research. However, national science policies cannot rest solely on these accidental occurences. There will frequently be areas of research identified as desirable but not yet established in a nation. There certainly are research problems especially relevant to given communities. In Australia and its territories, health of primitive peoples, harmful effects of sunlight on fair skins and long distance motor travel on bad roads are three examples that spring readily to mind. If a government wishes to get this kind of research off the ground, how can it do so?

In fact, this can rarely be done effectively by fiat. There are many examples of highly structured research systems, where priorities are set, projects conceived and implemented, through some central authority. These can work superbly well for technologic research, as the Manhattan project and the U.S. Space Programme have shown. However, this centralized approach does *not* work for basic research. The weakness of Soviet biological research and the mediocre quality of work in a number of mission-oriented U.S. government agencies provide abundant evidence of this. The really fundamental advances in biology and medicine come from individuals or small teams battling for prestige and funds in a free market system. Thus, the most effective way to get new research moving is by the use of ear-marked but still competitive research grant funds. A government, advised by its expert committees, can set up research professorships, special scholarships and grants for the field identified as important. This will gradually lure people, still motivated by free market forces, into the field. This type of fiscal weapon, wielded with restraint and mature judgement, can be most effective, and is certainly better than the setting up of yet another statutory authority or government institute, with all its inherent dangers of self-perpetuation.

*Further reading*

Himsworth H. and Delafresnaye J. F., eds., *The Support of Medical Research.* Blackwell Scientific Publications, Oxford (1956).

de Solla Price D. J., *Little Science, Big Science*, Columbia University Press, New York (1963).

Price D. K., *Government and Science: their dynamic relation in American democracy.* New York University Press (1954).

de Reuck A., Goldsmith M. and Knight J., eds., *Decision Making in National Science Policy. Ciba Foundation Symposium.* Little, Brown and Co. Boston (1968).

Weinberg A. M., *Reflections on Big Science.* The M.I.T. Press, Cambridge, Mass. (1967).

# 7

# Medical research and medical education

'*It is science that will provide the truly human basis of morals and politics in the future*'. Marcelin Berthelot (1901).

Universities have always been places of intellectual ferment and unrest. As they represent an important breeding ground for new ideas, and as social change rests on new ideas and attitudes, this is perfectly natural. However, it is doubtful whether the turmoil and revolt that pervaded universities between 1965 and 1970 has ever before been equalled, either in degree or in geographic spread. Although much of the noise was generated by professional or near-professional revolutionaries who simply used the university as a convenient vehicle or forum, one positive result of undoubted value has been a thorough re-examination by university academics themselves, of the role of the university in society. Indeed, such disaffection with universities as did exist amongst the more balanced and moderate students was not without foundation. One of the most commonly heard criticisms from this segment of the student body was that academics spent too much time and effort on research and too little on teaching. In this chapter, I hope to analyze the inter-relationships existing between research and education, and to answer the question of whether universities should be engaged in medical research at all. Lest the reader consider the point a little technical, let me reveal my aim in broaching the subject. Like many academics, I share Berthelot's hope (above), and consider the continuing and probable necessary struggle between 'town and gown' as a crucial one. To the extent that such struggles can be 'won', Berthelot's prediction depends on a victory for science and learning, or at least on a mutual resolution of the more outstanding problems between the academic world and society generally.

## Traditional role of universities

Traditionally, universities have been called upon to fulfil a triple role.

First, they must be living respositories of knowledge gathered during the past, staffed by experts who have mastered this knowledge. Secondly, they must be teaching institutions where knowledge is passed on to the younger generation in such a manner that continued learning, as a way of life, is encouraged. Thirdly, universities have been factories for new knowledge through research. The central question now is whether this third component is really necessary, or whether, especially in fields like biology and medicine, the universities should get out of research, leaving this to research institutes, thereby freeing more time for teaching.

Let us, therefore, look at the university's teaching role more closely. Few would deny that in medicine, much of the matter taught is subject to rapid change. In part this is because the concepts previously held have been shown to be wrong. More frequently, it is because a new discovery has placed the previously taught material into an entirely different perspective, thus necessitating a fundamental review of a subject's framework. Past experience suggest that this process of reassessment, review and change is a continuing one. There is little likelihood that discoveries will suddenly stop occurring. The graduate leaving a university must face the very real possibility that the store of knowledge garnered during his undergraduate course will gradually become superseded. The university teachers must therefore seek to inspire not only rote learning, but a balanced perspective in the minds of students. The student must be made to accept the material he is taught as the concensus reached by the world's best brains on that particular topic, but subject to later review. He must be encouraged to keep up to date in later life by reading and other forms of post-graduate education. It is evident that this kind of teaching places greater demands on the intellect of the teacher than does high school education. In fact, the teaching part of the job alone demands that university academics be people of high intelligence, maturity and judgement.

Turning to the allied non-research role of the university as a living repository of knowledge, it is clear that society needs to have access to the achievement and learning of the past. Much of this is embodied in the experts that staff universities. The degree to which the knowledge is integrated and filtered, or, as it were, stored in a creative way, will depend on the mental calibre of the people concerned.

The main point of the above analysis was to show that universities can only fulfil the first two traditional and vital roles if staffed by people of excellence. This brings us to the first and one of the strongest reasons for the need for continuing research in universities. As institutions, they must attract and hold extremely gifted men. It is a general, though by no means a universal, rule that men of this calibre will not be satisfied with teaching as a sole career outlet. Their creativity usually demands that they be given time to fulfil it in a direct way. This may be through reading and writing, but for most academics, it must needs be through research. Thus the need to preserve excellence in universities comes down to a need to preserve facilities for research.

I have said above that the general rule is not a universal one. Indeed, there is in universities a proportion of people who lead fulfilled and useful lives in teaching alone. These may be among the best teachers and almost certainly will be among those most popular with students. My point is *not* that these people should be discouraged – far from it. It is simply that if a university were to consist *solely* of this type of person, it would gradually go down hill. This is the next aspect which I wish to develop.

## Research as a spur to the updating of teaching

What I believe to be the crux of the problem is that teaching and research are inextricably intertwined, at least as far as the natural sciences are concerned. If we accept that what needs to be taught is subject to change, then we must ask how the university teacher can best encompass and master this change. An obvious reply would be that he should simply spend all his spare time reading the scientific literature. There are all kinds of practical reasons why this does not work. First, it is hard to master the literature as an outsider, and to find one's way through the morass of trivial and poor quality work to the key moving edges. Secondly, it is difficult to maintain perspective if the material being read is a cold, remote thing rather than something pertaining to one's own daily struggles in the laboratory. Thirdly, and most importantly, we must consider motivation. University dons are not saints, and the struggle to keep up is intensely demanding. If one is doing research, and getting a big proportion of his goal satisfaction from doing it effectively, there is a great spur to keeping on top of the literature. Without being aware of the major trends in bioscience, one simply cannot excel in research, and so the effective researcher will, when he teaches, give an up-to-date view – the same kind of current perspective as he needs and uses in his research. The pure teacher may well revamp his lectures extensively for the first few years, but there is a great danger of 'getting into a rut' if the intellectual atmosphere surrounding him is not pervaded with the ferment of change. The truly dedicated teacher may enjoy this ferment vicariously, and be sufficiently stimulated by research going on around him. Most people, however, seem to need that extra spur provided by their own involvement in research.

The reader may well, at this stage, have identified an objection to the above arguments. I have made it clear that research is highly specialized. Obviously a university man must teach many things other than the detailed subject of his researches. How, then, can his knowledge of this one strictly defined moving front help him in his much more general under graduate lectures? This objection is less powerful when one realizes the interdependence of the biosciences. A key change in orientation in one sub-speciality can cause significant ripples spreading far and wide through biology. Moreover, it must also be stressed that the teaching – research inter-action is a two-way one. The need to teach helps to keep interests general, and a general knowledge of biology makes specific research projects more enlightened and incisive. My claim, therefore, is that research helps teaching, and teaching helps research. This provides the second reason for keeping a major research effort within universities.

## Inter-relations between research institutes and universities

The third reason for maintaining research within universities relates to post-graduate education, which would be inconceivable if deprived of a research base. Here it is important that good human relationships exist between research institutes and the university with which they are most closely affiliated. Where these are present, the research institute can enhance the intellectual life of the university, and an involvement with the university can sharpen the work in the institute. Specifically, research institute staff can give occasional specialized lectures, which they enjoy doing, and which can have significant inspirational value; and university students can pursue their post-graduate studies partially or wholly in the research institute. It is not easy to achieve this good interaction, largely because the university man, torn between teaching, research and administration, tends to be jealous of his pure research counterpart.

A fourth and final reason justifying research in universities is that if all research were left to institutes, there might result a rather spotty coverage of the wide field of biological knowledge. Those disciplines which are prominent and important for the understanding of common diseases would have institutes devoted to them, but it would not be conceivable to visualize an institute for each of the 25 or so subjects comprising a medical curriculum. It may be that research in some of these fields will be pursued at a less intensive pace than in some others, and that for the most popular fields, research institutes will make the major contributions. This still leaves a vast area for university departments to cover, to the benefit of all mankind.

## Admission of a dilemma

I believe the foregoing arguments add up to an unanswerable case for the continuance of research as a major activity of universities. However, I admit that there is a dilemma in the present situation, where many of the best brains in universities really care very little about undergraduate education. I believe the answer to this dilemma lies in methods which enhance the prestige of teaching. More effort should be made by university administrations to monitor the effectiveness of teachers. Systems of student as well as colleague evaluation could be devised and tested for soundness and consistency. The task would not be an easy one, but no more difficult, after all, than the task of evaluation of research achievement. University committees would then be in a position to reward excellence in teaching by promotion, just as they now reward excellence in research. Moreover, one could consider devices such as prizes awarded for inspired teaching. Many kinds of research prizes now exist, worth little money but conferring prestige. A similar array for teaching, particularly for junior academics, could help substantially in creating a climate where a higher premium was placed on educational skills by academics themselves.

We have said much about how researchers learn their trade. It is a remarkable fact how little a university man is ever taught about the art and science of teaching. Of course, a big part of a gift for teaching lies in the genes; but there are many tricks that can formally be learnt. These include use of visual aids, speed of delivery, use of repetition, proper introductions to and summaries of lectures and many others. At the Hall Institute, we impress the importance of all these devices on budding researchers, just to improve efficiency of communications in research. How much more important that these be formally taught to the university teacher! Some exposure to a very practically-oriented course in educational methods should be obligatory for the would-be university lecturer.

## Continuing education as a way of life for clinicians

The primary concern of this book is medical research, and so we cannot explore in any great depth the important field of post-graduate medical education which could well be the subject of a book in its own right. Suffice it to make just two points. First, everything in the recent history of science suggests that patterns of medical investigation and treatment will continue to change as a result of further research discoveries. Secondly, few of these changes will constitute so dramatic an advance as to require immediate and total acceptance. In fact, the new drug or operation usually requires a prolonged period of critical evaluation before its real value can be assessed. The practising doctor is subjected to all sorts of pressures to move with the times. Pharmaceutical manufacturers bombard him with glossy publications, frequently written in pseudo-scientific terms, that laud the unique value of a new drug, which nine times out of ten is only marginally different from products that have been available for years. Patients often demand treatments that they have heard or read about. Even within the profession itself there is a certain desire to 'keep up with the Jones''. The only way that a practitioner can maintain a balanced outlook and can hope to distinguish between a real advance and a mere passing fashion is by accepting a commitment to continuing education. The discipline of consistent reading of the medical literature must be the cornerstone of this commitment. For example, it is amazing to what extent a weekly reading of just one journal, 'The Lancet', can keep one in touch with the moving front of internal medicine. Formal postgraduate courses are also important. In some countries, whole institutions are given over exclusively to post-graduate medical education. More frequently, post-graduate education is a rather loosely defined function of the university teaching hospital. For the most highly motivated doctors, this process of education never stops, and is aided by close affiliation with a major teaching centre.

From the practical viewpoint, postgraduate education aims to give the specialist the knowledge and skills needed to practice that specialty, and to ready him for the continuing process of dispassionate, objective evaluation of the results of treatment and of new procedures. It is in this latter process that a familiarity with research becomes very helpful. The physician who has done some research himself, or who has been closely associated with a research unit, is likely to be able to generate a higher standard of self-criticism. He will know a little of the methods by which conclusions have been reached, and he will have a greater sensitivity to the need for consulting technical experts about many matters of judgement. In contrast, doctors who have never had contact with research really know very little about its nature. They will find it more difficult to achieve a happy balance between never doing anything differently from when one was aged twenty-five and hopping onto each therapeutic bandwagon as it appears. Therefore a brief period in research can confer lasting benefit on a person whose future life will be entirely in practical medicine.

In the clinical sphere, postgraduate education and research are very closely linked. The budding specialist in neurology or orthopaedics receives most of his training on the job, taking progressively more senior resident and registrar positions in a large hospital. During these vital formative years, he will be closely involved with whatever research is going on in the department concerned. In many cases, he is required to spend two years or so in full-time research in order to gain his specialist qualification, though I would be reluctant to see this trend extended into geographical and conceptual spheres for which it is not yet relevant. At this stage of the world's development, it is not yet feasible for every clinician to have a period in research during his training. However, it is quite conceivable that in a more affluent and leisured world of the future, this might come to pass.

## Periodic Review of Licence to Practice

Some authorities are so convinced of the need for continuing education in medicine that they favour a system of periodic examination and review, whereby medical practitioners would be required to take an examination, e.g. each ten years, in order that their licence to practice be renewed. This viewpoint is idealistic and can be supported by strong arguments. Unquestionably the thought of an examination looming up would be a spur to study and self-review of performance. However, the proposal is quite unrealistic. It is difficult to see how one professional group could be made to examine itself in this way without the same principles applying to all professions. The cost would also be enormous, and who would undertake the job? In a free society, the national representatives of medicine would almost certainly refuse to do so. It is more realistic to campaign for increased standards within medical schools and increasingly demanding examinations by boards responsible for licencing of specialists. In many countries, a doctor only qualifies for specialist practice by passing a series of stringent examinations held 4 to 7 years after his initial graduation in medicine. One must then rely on his own integrity and motivation to provide the stimulus for maintenance of competence.

## Research exposure as a force to counteract drug promotion

Elsewhere in this book I have been at some pains to point out my admiration for much of the research that has been performed by the pharmaceutical industry. Not all the activities of this industry are equally admirable. One aspect that has been extensively criticized is the heavy expenditure on promotion, in particular by way of high-pressure detailers who visit general practitioners and provide them with elaborately prepared information describing the properties and benefits of new drugs. There are never untruths in these pamphlets or advertisements, but they do present evidence in a manner different from that of a technical article in a medical journal. Great skill goes into highlighting the most favourable aspect of the available evidence and literature. This form of promotion is highly effective. Many dispensing pharmacists claim that they can tell when a company's representative has been through a district by monitoring an increase in doctors' prescriptions for that company's drugs. The doctor who is able to read promotional literature critically and selectively, and to sift the available scientific evidence in a cold-blooded way uninfluenced by factors of pressure or personality, will be the one best able to help his patients. Much of the business of research deals with criticism of data and even self-criticism. A scientist must be a stern critic of his own objectivity and topic to forestall the criticism of his colleagues. It is the sharpening of this critical quality that may well be the most important legacy of a research apprenticeship. A physician who has spent a couple of years in the laboratory will be more sceptical than most about anecdotes praising this or that drug.

The fact is that three factors militate against easy assessment of a new drug's merit. First, many chronic diseases follow a waxing and waning course, and if therapy happens to coincide with one of the spontaneous upswings, it may appear to have done something marvellous. Secondly, there are great psychological factors in organic disease. A given physical injury or defect may appear trivial to a person with a stoical temperament, but may virtually disable a more sensitive or delicate person. Given this relation between psyche and soma, it is a frequent finding that the administration of therapy which a patient believes to be novel or special induces a feeling of well-being without there necessarily being any change in the patient's physical status. Thirdly, there is considerable individual variation in response to a drug. Patient A may truly benefit considerably more than patient B, usually for reasons that we are at a loss to understand. Therefore the assessment of the real place of a new drug by comparison with previous treatments of a disease is a long and difficult matter. It often requires a 'double-blind' controlled trial, an assessment process that John Rowan Wilson dramatized in his novel 'The Double Blind.'

In a double-blind controlled trial, as I mentioned briefly in Chapter 3, equal numbers of patients are randomly allocated into groups, one getting the new drug, the other either a dummy tablet with no drug content or else with some previously-accepted remedy in it. Neither the doctor nor the patient knows which individual is getting the new drug and which is not. This information is contained in a code which is only broken at the conclusion of the trial. The design of such trials is crucial, and involves consultations between physicians and statisticians even before the trial begins. The statistician helps the doctors to decide how many patients should be included in the trial, how long it should run, what objective measurements should be made to assess disease improvement, and so forth. In some trials, there are safeguards programmed in to ensure that if the drug is either dramatically better or dramatically worse than the dummy tablet, the code can be broken and the trial terminated. Unfortunately, real 'miracle' drugs are all too rare.

One would think that by now most doctors would be thoroughly familiar with the difficulties of objective assessment of therapy. Remarkably enough, however, many doctors are still believers in 'anecdotal medicine'. There is an immediacy to one's own personal experience that may transcend logic, and if the first patient for whom one has personally prescribed drug A derives striking benefit, one may be tempted to go on prescribing it come what may. There is perhaps also a psychological need in doctors to believe very firmly in what they are doing. Such belief in one's own wisdom and power may even be of positive benefit to the patient in some circumstances. Nevertheless, we must increasingly move from anecdotal medicine to scientific medicine, and this will become progressively easier as more doctors become familiar with research philosophy and methods.

## Medical education and the developing nations

So far in this book, we have been considering the impact of research on medicine as practiced in affluent societies. Over three-quarters of the world's population does not yet have access to the kind of medical care that the reader has come to accept as commonplace. We must now consider some of the problems of medical education and research in the less affluent communities.

There is no doubt that so much medical knowledge already exists as to revolutionize health in developing nations, could it but be applied to the large numbers of people involved. It is therefore frequently argued that new research is just not relevant to these nations. This argument is false, for a number of reasons which are a little subtle. All of them, one way or another, relate to the need to keep gifted people working in their own nations.

Let us deal first with the staffing of medical schools. An abbreviated medical course, with more emphasis on pragmatic medicine than on theoretical foundations, will usually be the sensible compromise reached during the initial years of such institutions. Nevertheless, the schools will still only be as good as the men that staff them. There is no question that people with outstandingly good brains emerge with sufficient frequency in less developed nations. Frequently, these gifted men and women sincerely want to help their country get on its feet. As part of the natural pilgrim's progress, such would-be leaders currently spend a few years working in some major centre in the European world, the notable exception being leaders from China. It is not unusual for the scholar from Asia, Africa or South America to attract notice because of his intelligence and industry, and to be offered considerable inducements to stay in the United States, Canada, Sweden or wherever it may be. If no institutional framework exists to allow the person some outlet for creativity in his own country, the temptation to stay abroad may become insuperable. Therefore, there should be some opportunity for research in even the humblest, most practical of medical schools. This need not involve approaches as sophisticated and demanding of equipment and money as are usual in Western countries. Problems abound that require chiefly intelligence, time, opportunity and ingenuity. It is saddening to note how frequently not even minimal facilities for research are available.

A second factor relates to the rate of emergence of nations from underdeveloped status. Even a superficial look at Japan, Thailand, Singapore and Hong Kong over the past few decades proves how rapid this can be. Such emerging nations will clamour for high standards of health care and a rapid rate of progress in health consistent with the newly-won affluence. Again, the necessary institutional framework will not appear overnight. A nation that wants Western-style medical care in 50 years time must *today* begin to motivate the most gifted individuals patiently and progressively to build that framework and to foster traditions of academic thinking and excellence. A local research base would help materially.

The geographic variability of human disease incidence represents a third reason why less affluent nations should become involved in research. Many serious infections and parasitic diseases occur only in tropical zones. Some cancers are 100 times more common in certain locations than elsewhere, frequently for reasons that are quite unknown. The research necessary to uncover the reasons and to control the causes must be done locally. At present, the main burden of such research falls on international organizations, for example the World Health Organization, or on individual investigators who have developed an interest in epidemiology, anthropology, geographical pathology or some such field. Excellent though such research may be, the end result is that there is far less work being done on disease problems of the underdeveloped world than on those of affluent communities. Governments are much more generous with respect to research that may benefit the tax-payer than for research sponsored for wider humanitarian motives. Thus a better research base in the underdeveloped world might be necessary before many of these problems are effectively tackled.

Over the past decade or so I have detected a healthy shift in the directions that official thinking is taking with respect to sponsorship of research in the third world. The old pattern was to take young doctors and scientists from the less affluent nation and bring them to the West for advanced training. The new thinking reverses the process. Experts from the Western world are brought to the developing country and set up research training programmes right in the local setting. The young worker does not suffer the cultural dislocation of a move to the west, and does not develop a desire for complex equipment and support as he would if sent to Harvard, Stanford or Cambridge. In turn, the western scientist doing the training comes to understand the local problems and adapts the level and direction of his programme accordingly. It is, of course, desirable that the initiative for maintaining the programme is, sooner or later, assumed by nationals of the country concerned. It is also clear that travel and development of a world perspective can benefit a would-be scientist, from whatever nation. However, this is less likely to be accompanied by a desire to escape from local responsibilities if the person is more mature and already invested with some seniority in his own home base.

An interesting example of this new type of research training centre concept is provided in my own field of immunology. The World Health Organization sponsors a series of Immunology Research and Training Centres (IRTC) in countries such as Nigeria, Singapore, Brazil and India. These have two allied functions: to give courses in modern immunology and its role in medicine; and to provide a research laboratory designed to act as a focal point for local initiatives in the field. Typically, only one or two staff members will be westerners, and the enterprise runs on a minimal WHO-sponsored budget supplemented by whatever funds the investigators can raise from elsewhere. The work of the IRTC is performed by these staff members aided by visiting lecturers drawn from all over the world, and, with increasing frequency, by young people from the host nation itself. Both the training and the research places special emphasis on local problems. Thus, the Singapore centre currently focusses its research on nasopharyngeal carcinoma, a cancer at the back of the throat. This is exceptionally frequent amongst Chinese, and there is some evidence of association with a particular virus, the so-called EB virus, which causes different diseases in people of differing genetic constitutions. While the training in immunology that students receive is, of course, much wider, there is still a conscious bias towards diseases such as leprosy or parasitic infestations, of special local importance. It is perhaps too early to tell what impact these IRTC will have on the development of medical science in the host countries, but I should be most surprised if they do not turn out to represent a very astute investment.

*Further reading*

G. Wolstenholme and M. O'Connor, eds., *Teamwork for World Health. Ciba Foundation Symposium.* J. and A. Churchill, London (1971).

J. M. Ziman, *Public Knowledge. An essay concerning the social dimension of science.* Cambridge University Press (1968).

# 8

# Medical science and the layman

'*Knowledge of the physicochemical determinants of life is of course essential for the understanding of man's nature*'. R. Dubos

Most readers will at some time have had occasion to walk into a room filled with people all belonging to a specialist group. Be they surgeons, engineers, lawyers, racing-car drivers or farmers, it can be a discomforting experience. The intruder interrupts a flow of communication that is dependent on special knowledge, shared commitment, and, frequently, a shorthand language or jargon peculiar to that group. The professional link creates a certain cosiness of relationship, an atmosphere where each member of the group is sure of his place and comfortable in the knowledge of a commonality that does not require explicit expression. Often the group welcomes the outsider into the discussion, only to find that the attempts to communicate with him, to bring him into the circle, are so slow and clumsy as to destroy the atmosphere. Nowhere is this subculture problem more marked than in communication between scientist and layman.

It is a truism to say that modern society has over the last century been reshaped more by science and technology than by any other factor. Equally, it is clear that many people are bewildered and upset by the unwanted side-products of a technical society-congestion, pollution, possibility of mass destruction, and so forth. This can lead non-scientists to mistrust and fear science, and can widen the split between scientist and layman. In this chapter, I shall attempt to analyze how this formidable cultural barrier can be overcome. I believe the problem is an urgent one, and capable of solution if attacked with energy and goodwill.

### Scientists and secondary education

A logical entry point for discussion, though one relevant only to the long term, is the nature and quality of science teaching in secondary schools. My impression is that this has improved tremendously over the last 20 years, with partial breakdown of rigid disciplinary compartmentation, increased use of attractive illustrations in books, and greater emphasis on and facilities for laboratory and field work. There is still room for expansion of one particular kind of teaching aid, and that is the use of film. A well-made science film combines the best features of lecture and textbook. It can engage the child's imagination by featuring a personality, perhaps one of the world's great scientists in the field under study. It can have significant visual content, be this by way of charts or diagrams, or examples of primary data, such as microscopic photographs or views of the stars through a powerful telescope. It can detail actual experimental manipulations and give glimpses into the nature of research. Perhaps most important of all, it has the potential for extraordinarily wide dissemination of information. The scientist who gives an hour-long talk to a group of school children has invested, say, three hours of his time to communicate his points to an audience of say, 30 to 300 children. The scientist who prepares an outstanding film on his subject may invest 100 hours of his time, plus the time of many others, into the venture. However, he then has a vehicle which could reach literally millions of children over a span of several years.

It is clear that there will always be a time-gap between a discovery and its impact on science education in schools. However, it is important that this gap be minimized as far as practical. Students will become disenchanted if their classroom work falls too far behind what they read in *Life* magazine or see on popular science television. Established scientists can help here by taking an active role in the preparation of school text books. They may not find the time to do the primary job of writing the book, but should hold themselves available for reviewing the segment thereof relevant to their own subject, and, where necessary, replacing outmoded concepts with new ones. There have been some exciting ventures in this field in Australia in recent years, with prominent scientists playing a leading role in the production of really outstanding textbooks and no doubt the same is true in other countries. It will be interesting to see if, 20 years hence, the decision-makers trained in science according to these modern techniques possess a better grip of science and its methods as a result.

In Sydney, Australia, Professor Harry Messel has been instrumental in instigating a creative experiment in science education for outstanding youngsters. Each year, he runs an international science school for two weeks in his Department of Physics of the University of Sydney. The faculty consists of about six of the world's leading scientists in the field of study chosen for the year; this is frequently in the physical sciences but, on occasion, a biology course is given instead. The students consist of highly selected 16 to 17 year old school children from all over Australia, about 100 all told, together with 20 scholars from the United States, the United Kingdom and Japan. Beyond any facts that the teenagers may learn, there is an important inspirational element in the exercise. The students are exposed to great minds at an impressionable age. Moreover, they meet and mix with exceptionally gifted members of their own peer group drawn from a wide geographic spectrum. It is likely that a good proportion of the students are marked for life by this early experience. In the United Kingdom, the BBC programme 'Young Scientist of the Year' has clearly proved of considerable value in promoting an interest in original scientific work in schools.

## Scientists and the mass media

Secondary and tertiary education dictate the broad pattern of a person's life interests, and subsequent additions to knowledge come from many quarters. However, it is obvious that the mass media play a big role in shaping public knowledge and attitudes. This is a continuing process, lasting throughout life, and because of this may even over-ride formal education as the prime source of usable knowledge. Newspapers, magazines, radio and television – each in their own way are vitally important in both mirroring and shaping society.

All in all, the relationship between scientists and the mass media is an uneasy one. We are living in an age of instant communications and information explosion. The mass media are at their best when covering the spectacular, the immediate, the obvious. Dealing with a landing on the moon, a political crisis, a natural disaster, the media come into their own. They are much less geared to the subtle, the qualified, the unglamorous norms of social progress. Yet the bulk of modern science is of this ilk. The dramatic breakthrough that journalists love to predict or to create is almost always chimaeric. Individual events in science are rarely the stuff of which newspaper headlines are made, though the summation of these events may dominate history.

This being the case, scientists and the media often face one another with mutual mistrust. The scientist is impatient with the journalist's desire for a catchy simplification or an immediate human application. The journalist is irritated by the scientist's desire to qualify and equivocate, and by his escape into incomprehensible jargon. The outcome of the confrontation is frequently unsatisfactory to both.

## Room for improvement in attitudes and performance of scientists

There is a need for reappraisal from both sides of the fence, and in fact there is much that can be done to improve the situation. A large part of the blame lies with the scientist himself. He is, after all, a rather privileged person. He is paid by society to do work that vitally interests him; he has an extraordinary degree of personal freedom and self-determination; he is amongst the few elements in society who, like an artist or an athlete, sets his own boundary conditions rather than having them imposed from outside; unlike the artist or athlete, he is usually well-paid and secure without necessarily being a world-beater. In other words, it could be argued that the scientist owes it to society to account for his activities and to justify his privileged status. One way in which he can discharge this debt is to make a bigger effort to communicate his discoveries in language understandable by laymen.

Many scientists bluntly refuse to have anything to do with the media, and look with suspicion on their colleagues who feature frequently on television or in the newspapers. The latter are dismissed as publicity-seekers or blowhards. Such a reluctance to step into the limelight is often accompanied by an exaggerated fear of misrepresentation. The scientist may give as his reason for refusing to be interviewed the excuse that 'journalists never get it right'. I have found that, with a little patience and effort, a scientific discovery can be put into a form interesting to ordinary people. This usually demands some over-simplification and avoidance of the qualifying, modifying phraseology of which scientists are so fond. Moreover, one cannot readily assign proper credit to all the other scientists who made antecedent discoveries in the field, as one would in a formal scientific paper. The different medium demands a different attitude and different techniques. Apart from a little gentle ribbing by my colleagues, most reactions to my own efforts to popularize science, particularly Australian achievements in science, have been reasonably favourable. Thus I feel that the erosion of status resulting from responsible communication with the media which many scientists fear is largely an illusion.

Scientists anxious to keep the public informed should be aware of the considerable effort involved. The radio talk, newspaper article or television interview may well require more preparation and checking than a routine technical paper. It is vital to remember the total absence of relevant background knowledge in the audience, and to build this up gradually before coming to the newest discovery. Wherever possible, the finished product should be checked for inaccuracies that may have crept in. Effort is required to maintain an atmosphere that is sober and responsible rather than sensationalistic. Journalists anxious to pin one down about 'cancer cures', 'break-throughs', or predictions about the likely timing of a discovery not yet on the horizon, must be dealt with politely but firmly. Given this extra effort, communication between scientist and layman can be useful as well as good fun. The need to place the work into broad perspective can even help the scientist to see himself and his field more clearly.

## Role of science journalism

The media in their turn can improve their role in communication between scientist and non-scientist. The first pre-requisite is a realization that science reporting is specialized – just as specialized as financial or political reporting, or more so. The larger and more responsible components of the media have realised this, but one way or another a big part of the world's science reporting is still done by totally untrained personnel. The second element is a need to avoid exaggeration. The temptation, particularly in the medical field, is great. It must be resisted, however, because a false alarm concerning some new treatment for a disease creates a great deal of unnecessary human distress. A third realization that would help the media is that people are interested in things even if they are not immediately useful. In describing an area of biological research, it is easy to slip into a mode that presupposes the only interest of the work to be its eventual relevance to cancer or some other disease. However, there is a big part of man's nature that just wants to know and is thrilled by a new insight purely for its own sake. There should be more effort to develop this side of the public's consciousness. It is, after all, the side that provides motivation and joy for the scientist himself, and this should be shared with society.

In general terms, I have found that science is more suitable for treatment as feature material than as news. There are some outstandingly good examples of science journalism using the more leisurely, digested approach suitable for features or documentaries. When science is treated as news, strange things can happen. First, sub-editors compose headlines and dissect copy. I have not infrequently been in the position where some rather technical advance was discussed at a public lecture, but where the next day's headlines read 'breakthrough in multiple sclerosis' or 'leukaemia vaccine in sight'. Interestingly, the report under that headline was often reasonably accurate and the headline itself the main offender. This indicates that editorial staff may need more education than science reporters!

Secondly, science achievements treated as news material are frequently picked up by the big international wire services (Reuters, A. P., etc), and the end result is a degree of exposure quite inconsistent with either the intentions of the scientist or the importance of the new discovery. It can happen that a fairly routine interview with a young reporter, in which he is given research information appropriate for strictly local public relations purposes, fires the young man's imagination and causes him to word his article injudiciously. The non-existing breakthrough could, next morning, be headline news from San Francisco to Istanbul! This sounds far-fetched, but it has happened in my own institution, needless to say to the great embarrassment of all concerned. Of course, there are occasions when a scientific discovery is of world shaking importance, but these are rare indeed compared to those where scientists reveal results of considerable but still limited interest.

One way by which journalistic inaccuracies can be eliminated is for scientists to write more feature articles under their own name. This is happening to an increasing extent, and several famous scientists actually write a weekly column. Perhaps some mechanism could be envisaged by which leading scientists were actively urged by their own learned societies to write one newspaper article per year. This would provide the public with much authoritative information, and would not place an excessive burden on any individual. Periodic authoritative and responsible releases from universities and research institutes also play a valuable role in the overall journalistic process.

Television is a medium uniquely suited to good science journalism. Most science documentaries made for television that I have seen have been of real value. However, the volume of science television is still small in most countries. Clearly a television science programme will be more expensive to produce than a radio programme of broadly similar content, but the former is likely to be more informative with the added visual content, and thus likely to reach a much bigger audience. I would welcome a greatly expanded effort by the television networks in the science field.

## Layman's attitude to scientific information

So far, we have examined the problem of communication largely from the points of view of scientists and journalists. What of the layman himself? His attitude and overall willingness to learn more about science is at least equally important. It is a pity that many people consider popular science rather like a dose of medicine – good for you but somewhat unpleasant.

Unfortunately, many popular science presentations, particularly oral ones, take place in a setting that evokes a certain schoolroom atmosphere. As soon as this creeps in, two factors appear: boredom and exaggerated respect for the superior knowledge of the expert. Popular science should be interesting and vital, non-dogmatic, and, where possible, a little controversial. Discussion periods or other forms of audience participation should be encouraged. In this way, the intelligent layman is made to feel a partner in the exercise.

The point has frequently been made that scientists appreciate music, art, literature and other humanities; but that humanists fail to adopt a similar attitude to science. The fact is that both aspects of culture can enrich the life of everyone, and one cannot lay claim to being educated without an acquaintance with each side. The person who ignores science is simply not living in the real world. An honest striving for understanding of broad trends and goals in science will create citizens better fitted for the present rapidly changing era.

## Public discussion of socio-scientific issues

There are many major issues on the political scene that have a strong science component. Building dams or nuclear power stations, spending more on defence or hospitals, subsidizing industries or taxing them, decentralizing industry or curbing pollution; all of these require political decisions that can only be made competently if based on suitable advice concerning their scientific aspects. Frequently, governments rely for such advice on a small nucleus of senior scientists in their own employ. These individuals, valuable though they may be, cannot possibly be expert in everything. Many of these issues would benefit from a period of wide public discussion in which a nation's scientists could contribute their views both as experts in the field and as citizens. This constitutes yet one more reason why scientists must descend from their ivory tower and assume their full social responsibilities. There are so many decisions which must be made in a free society to which the scientist holds a vital key. He must not always remain neutral. If the decision must be taken at a particular time, it is no use his proclaiming that all the evidence is not in, and that two more years research are necessary. Frequently, history will not wait. If he holds back from controversy, decisions will be taken by others, perhaps on the basis of less informed judgments. The proper course for the scientist to take is to form a view on the balance of probabilities as he sees them, and to express that view in an appropriate forum.

## Public appreciation of fundamental versus applied science

It requires considerable effort to understand the nexus relationship between fundamental science and applied science. When science is under attack by laymen, as it is at the present time, it is frequently fundamental research at which this attack is directed. Few would associate themselves directly with a plea for diminution in research aimed at a cancer cure or a safer motor car, but the academic engaged in long range fundamental research makes an easy target. This is somewhat ironic, as pure research probably accounts for less than ten percent of global expenditure on research and development. The bulk of the funds goes towards scientific work aimed at clearly defined practical objectives. We are always in danger of oversimplification, and few aspects of this are more irritating than the catch cry of 'relevance' in research. Is it more 'relevant' to spend hundreds of millions of dollars screening through several thousand more organic chemicals with possible anti-cancer activity, employing some highly artificial mouse model, than to engage in fundamental research in cell biology that might open a whole new vista in the cancer field? Any command that all research must have an immediate pay-off would, if obeyed, signal an end to real scientific revolutions. Perhaps the most important message of this book is the inter-relatedness of scientific progress, but public understanding of this is still at a primitive level.

The difficulties inherent in explaining the value of fundamental science to laymen are not insuperable. It is no longer sufficient to dodge the issue and pretend that all biological research, for example, is a form of cancer research. What is required is a patient analysis, illustrated by striking examples, of the dependence of applied research on a base of pure science. Furthermore, the scientist's own need to find a creative outlet in 'knowledge for knowledge's sake' should be frankly admitted, and not disguised as some vague hope for future practical benefits for society. In the last analysis, the decision of how much scientific research there should be in a country is a political one. The level achieved is a consequence of a national concensus reached about the importance of research. It would be neither feasible nor proper for scientists alone to determine the level. The concensus eventually reached will, however, be a much more enlightened one if the information that community leaders and the public generally possess about science is more accurate and extensive.

## Personal contacts between scientists and community leaders

Because of the difficulties of subcultures, with their own jargons and their own self-reinforcing sources of ego satisfaction, there is not as much personal contact as there should be between the leaders of various aspects of a country's life. Specifically, scientists tend to have little respect for politicians and rarely go out of their way to seek them out. This is true, though to a lesser extent, for the attitude of scientists towards the business and commercial world. All too frequently, when personal contacts between scientist and community leader do occur, it is in a setting of confrontation. The scientist approaches his political masters or the industrial giant with a specific proposal. Usually it is a request for funds or a representation on behalf of some vested interest. I would like to see more personal contacts in a neutral setting, where scientist meets politician essentially to explain the background and nature of his scientific work, and to receive feedback from the politician as to what the public really feels about science. I have experienced many examples of how a personal, neutral occasion of the above sort, accompanied by some simple demonstration of a new laboratory phenomenon, has provided a surprising degree of interest and pleasure for a non-scientific visitor. Such occasions may in fact, do more to shape his attitude to science than voluminous technical reports. Wide adoption of a policy where science leaders consciously set themselves the goal of regularly making these contacts could result in a ground-swell of enthusiasm for science within a few years.

There is a justifiable degree of indecision within science itself about the extent to which it should become enmeshed in activities such as public relations and lobbying. Aspects of this are very foreign to the scientific way of thinking. However, two factors suggest to me that organized science needs to be active, at least to a degree, in these fields. The first is that if pressure does not come from a central, responsible source, it will certainly come from individual interested parties. Frequently the individual scientist who pushes hard on behalf of his project, his institution or his subject is not the one with the greatest ability or foresight in that field. Secondly, scientific research is a big drain on the public purse and will increasingly be called on to defend its *raison d'etre*. It may be as well for the science establishment in various countries to consider in some detail the lines of communication between science and officialdom.

### The layman and medical science

Medical science occupies a special place in this discussion as, to a greater or lesser degree, *all* laymen are interested in health, at least their own and that of their families. While this puts the medical scientist at some advantage with respect of his counterpart in, for example, the physical sciences, it also imposes a need for responsibility and restraint. It is most important not to take advantage of people's natural fears. It frequently happens that someone wishes to give a large sum of money to my Institute because the individual or a close relative suffers from some severe disease. I deem it especially important to point out to such people the true relationship of our ongoing research programmes to progress in understanding of their particular condition. Frequently, such honest discussion confirms their resolve to help medical research, and on occasion they must be referred on to a scientist elsewhere engaged in more relevant research. In the long run, an equally open approach is also the best policy vis-a-vis governments, foundations and others involved in medical research support.

As regards the mass media, their chief focus of interest tends to be on health delivery rather than health research. There is a clear and important place for journalistic coverage of topics like hospital finances, health insurance schemes, consumption of pharmaceutical products, approaches to geriatric medicine and the like. Great popularity also attaches to the 'doctor who tells' type column, where currently available treatments of human diseases are discussed. Though many of these endeavours are in very bad taste, others fulfil a real educational role. When we move to research, I fear the great tendency is for over-sensationalistic coverage. As one deeply immersed in fundamental research in transplantation biology, I am acutely aware of this point, and must admit that the blame does not always lie with the journalists alone. There is probably no way that lurid coverage of medical research can be avoided. The best one can hope for is that the more serious newspapers give the lead in setting a dignified tone. This is certainly the case already for many publications. For example, coverage of medicine in the 'New York Times' is remarkably balanced and informative, and in fact to be written up there is deemed a source of prestige by many scientists! As the public becomes better informed about medical research, it may gradually become more aware of both the strengths and the limitations of medical science. If so, I believe both society and the medical profession would benefit. The doctor has far too long been regarded as an omnipotent 'little tin god' by some segments of society. The fact that this attitude is disappearing and is being replaced by a more realistic one can only be welcomed by all thinking people.

## The science subculture and public mores

Let us turn now to a much more subtle effect of science on the layman, one which is at once a source of difficulty and a source of strength. In the science subculture, it has long been evident that truth and honesty pay handsome personal dividends. There have been occasions where scientists have faked laboratory results, and in the short term, have gained notoriety as a consequence. However, the very essence of science is reproducibility. If a finding cannot readily be reproduced by laboratories other than that of the discoverer, it can suffer only one of two fates. Either it is formally discredited, usually through someone spotting an honest fault in experimental design or interpretation; or it is quietly forgotten. In neither case does the irreproducible finding hold a place in the expanding fabric of science. This being the case, there is no long-term advantage for the scientist who fabricates results or who in any way exaggerates or misrepresents his observed data. Prestige and rewards accrue only to the consistent contributor to the growing, shifting framework.

Scientists are not saints, and there is plenty of room in science for showmanship, salesmanship, gamesmanship and so forth. Nevertheless there is a basic undercurrent of honesty and openness that is a central feature of the scientific life. In the vast majority of cases, the fruits of one's life's labour are freely given away. The research results that are the only 'saleable product' of the scientist are either presented at an open meeting or published in a technical journal, and from that moment on, they are public property. In medical science, with the exception of research done by the pharmaceutical industry, patenting of discoveries is quite rare. The whole system of sanctions and rewards is quite different from that pertaining in industry.

The difficulty that this creates is at the level of communication. Many laymen who have 'come up the hard way' in a free enterprise system simply cannot understand or believe this way of life; or else they reach the view that academics are incredibly naive. I am not implying that business men are always crooked, devious or slavishly self-interested. I am aware that, in big business particularly, the motive and ideal of public service is challenging the profit motive as the number one driving force. Nevertheless, industry and commerce represent tougher schools and fundamentally different subculture systems. A different spectrum of human activities and attributes is valued and rewarded, and personal relationships are built on a different basis. Until this is more fully analyzed and better appreciated, there will always be a certain communications gap between scientist and layman.

In what respect is the concept of rigid honesty in science a source of strength for society? This lies in the gradual permeation of the view that truth pays, honesty pays. Fundamentally I believe this to be true in every walk of life, business and politics included, but it is somehow more obviously and transparently the case in science. As society is increasingly shaped by science, so the mores of the science subculture infiltrate themselves further into public mores. Jacob Bronowski has developed this point extensively. He claims that the great ethical force of science has been the dissemination of the idea that truth is a thing which will, in some way, help us all. Science has made us recognize that it is easier to run a society made up of independent individuals if they all acknowledge what is true.

## Science, orthodoxy and tolerance

The questioning spirit of science is another strong cultural force. Many non-scientists lead their lives according to some fixed set of beliefs that is so integral to their personalities as to be beyond possibility of questioning. Scientists have as their job the constant task of challenging orthodoxy, and of replacing concepts and laws when new experimental data show the established way of looking at things to be outmoded. Science is thus basically anti-authoritarian, and, to a certain extent, pragmatic. It is not entirely clear to me to what extent these attitudes spread from the professional lives of scientists into their personal lives. There is obviously much heterogeneity, and a contribution by childhood, social and national influences. However, from a statistical viewpoint, there will be a preponderance of scientists adopting liberal, humanist agnostic positions rather than conservative, dogmatically religious ones. It could well be argued that science has been one of the forces impelling the world gradually to the left.

In much of his work, the scientist moves from uncertainty to uncertainty. He must constantly draw general inferences from particular observations. While he seeks certitude and accuracy in the observation, he will often be tentative about its real place in the overall scheme of things. He spawns facts but gropes for meanings. One product of this way of life is tolerance. He becomes aware that other people, confronted with the same observations, place these into a different framework, possibly even reaching opposite conclusions. He comes to see this as their right, and, if he is a good scientist, he is prepared to change his mind and admit his errors. Working in an atmosphere of this kind, it is difficult not to extend this tolerance into other aspects of one's life. The longer one is a scientist, the more the prejudices which each of us brings with us into adulthood drop away. This diminution of prejudice is accelerated by international travel. Prominent scientists are exceedingly fortunate in being required to travel widely, and, I believe, play a major role in promoting international understanding and tolerance. Moreover, their friends, students and professional contacts share vicariously in the mellowing process. In fact, scientists are so used to thinking in international terms that the prospect of some stable form of world government seems less impossible to them than to others. The whole burden of this chapter has been the hope that the scientist and his views will permeate into the social fabric. If this happens, society would indubitably become more tolerant as a result.

I believe deeply that communication between scientist and layman is important. Now, more than ever before, life is what we make it. The meaning of life is the meaning which we consciously care to give it. The great causes shaping the direction of society are those which we identify and espouse. Our power to eradicate the historic evils of pestilence, famine, poverty and ignorance, while not infinite, is yet vastly greater than it was even 50 years before. Overpopulation, war, abuse of natural resources and man-made deterioration of the environment remain as threats to the human species. If these are to be overcome at all, it can only be through the better application of science and technology. If we forswear more science and technology, we cannot solve the problems that science and technology have brought us. If man's fate is left to chance, hundreds of millions may die as a result. Herein lies the central motive behind this book. Scientists and laymen must find a common language.

*Further reading*

Bronowski J., *Science and Human Values*. J. Messner, New York (1956).
Conant J. B., *On Understanding Science: an historical approach*. Yale University Press, New Haven (1947).
Dubos R. J., *The Dreams of Reason: Science and Utopias*. Columbia University Press, New York (1961).
Dubos R. J., *Reason Awake: Science for Man*. Columbia University Press, New York (1970).

# 9

# Medical research and advances in treatment of disease

'*It would be absurd to suppose that the explosive power of science is exhausted, or has even reached its maximum*'. Bertrand Russell

Most thinking people have, at some time, asked themselves whether medical science will ever produce weapons against cancer, heart disease or mental illness as dramatically and self-evidently effective as the antibiotics have been in the field of infections. In all these great problem areas of medicine, progress is being made, but no panacea is in immediate sight. The way is thus open for any pundit or would-be soothsayer to make whatever predictions he wishes, and these range from gloomiest pessimism to science-fictional, unrealistic optimism. From all I have said of the process of discovery, the reader will realize that the whole history of science proves that one can *not* forecast what is around the corner. As recently as 1933, Lord Rutherford ridiculed the notion of practical applications of nuclear power; the gap to Hiroshima was just 12 years. In this chapter, I will attempt to avoid posing as a visionary. I will, however, try to dissect the nature of the practical achievements in scientific medicine so far, and to use my knowledge of research in one restricted field of medicine, namely immunology, to make some reasonable predictions about relevant medical advances over the next ten to fifteen years. This may help the reader in developing a better perspective towards the voluminous amount of subject matter on this topic to which he will inevitably be exposed over the years.

### Analysis of major achievements in the health field

Health status and life expectancy have changed dramatically in the developed world over the last two hundred years. The advances that have achieved this improvement can be considered under four headings, namely social factors, preventive medicine, medicine and surgery. The social factors are doubtless the most important contributors from a statistical viewpoint. Efficient sewage disposal, greater emphasis on personal cleanliness, better housing with less overcrowding and more balanced nutrition have had major influence. These are in no sense medical achievements, but as the industrial revolution was made possible by applied science, one can justly claim that, at least indirectly, these social changes were helped by scientific research.

Preventive medicine is an important, expanding field and can boast of many triumphs. The greatest of these is mass immunization against epidemic diseases. The virtual eradication from the Western world of smallpox, diphtheria, typhoid fever, whooping cough, tetanus and poliomyelitis is due in large measure to 70 years of medical research in immunology since Pasteur, and to enlightened public health administration. An interesting contributing factor is the concept of 'herd immunity.' For a virulent micro-organism to survive and thrive, it must find a suitable population or density of susceptible hosts. Once a significant proportion of the population, e.g. 70 per cent, is immune, many epidemics are found not to be able to 'get off the ground', and so the immune status of the 70 per cent confers a certain degree of protection on the 30 per cent that are non-immune. This is, of course, no excuse for laxity in immunization programmes. There are still quite a number of infections for which no suitable vaccine exists, and we shall look at likely progress later in this chapter.

Many other public health and preventive medicine measures, less dramatic fruits of scientific medicine, must be considered. The discovery of the importance of vitamins accelerated the trend to better nutrition and gave it a scientific basis. Education and screening programmes have helped towards earlier diagnosis and hence better treatment of diseases like tuberculosis, venereal disease and some forms of cancer. The hygienic aspects referred to above have been placed on a formal footing, with monitoring of many aspects of the domestic and industrial environment. Many countries have made efforts towards routine medical examination of schoolchildren, with a view to picking up both physical and mental diseases at early, remediable stages. We will examine in detail the question of how far this pattern of routine health screening should be extended in the future.

## Surgery and surgical sub-specialties

There is continuous friendly rivalry between the two main branches of medical practice, medicine and surgery. Surgeons argue that their swift, technical approach leads to definite problem resolution, while the physician only stems the tide, treating symptoms and not causes. Physicians respond that most disease problems are not localized to one anatomical region but reflect subtler and wider abnormalities than the surgeon can deal with. I might add that neither side would argue the point too strongly, and in actual practice there is a great deal of collaboration between the two camps. In hospital medicine, in particular, elaborate effort goes into maintaining dialogue both with respect to disease in general and to the individual patient. The division does concern us here, as the two branches have contributed in different ways to the advanced point which we have reached in health care.

Surgery unquestionably has triumphed in the field of trauma, aided, of course, by antibiotics and other medical treatments. Important surgical sub-specialties such as plastic and reconstructive surgery, orthopaedics and neurosurgery have emerged. They are playing a large part in repairing the damage done by dangerous driving, wars, industrial accidents and other hazards of modern life, each having other roles as well. Surgery is frequently the most successful way of dealing with sudden emergencies resulting from disease. Few could quarrel with the surgeon's dominance when an internal organ (appendix, stomach) suddenly springs a leak, or when a hernia will not go back because a loop of bowel has wormed its way into it and cannot slip out. In these situations, the possibilities for a swift, definitive and often final solution of the problem are good.

There are other fields in which surgical progress has been only fair. This applies in many forms of cancer. Some cancers have spread imperceptibly from their site of origin even when the primary focus is still of very small size. When the lump is first noticed or the unexplained bleeding, hoarseness or cough leads to diagnosis, the surgeon may be able to remove the obvious cancer, only to see the microscopic satellite deposits later grow and spread further. It is important to avoid undue pessimism here. Many cancers are cured by surgery, and medical treatment of some others is improving. However, surgery could not be considered the final answer to cancer. Peptic ulcers are being operated on less frequently now than previously, and the trend is for less extensive operations, as removal of a large part of the stomach has been found to lead to many complications. Partial blockages of blood vessels or other internal tubes makes much work for modern surgeons. Here again, the contribution is frequently life-saving in an immediate sense but the eventual outcome may be clouded by a continuation, after surgery, of the disease process that caused the blood clot or the gall stone in the first place. In other words, more frequently than is generally realized, the surgeon is not the olympian arbiter between life and death, but simply one contributor in the continuing battle between the medical profession and a patient's illness.

Specialization has reached an advanced degree in surgery. The existence of specialists that deal with eyes, ear, nose and throat, or gynaecological problems is well known. What is less well recognized is that within what used to be termed general surgery, there is now extensive division of labour. There are thoracic surgeons versus abdominal surgeons; vascular surgeons versus biliary surgeons, and so forth. This process of development of special knowledge and skills is virtually limitless. Thus, amongst a group of plastic surgeons working at a large hospital, one may develop a deeper commitment to hand surgery, another to head and neck work, a third towards cosmetic repairs. This ultra-specialization within a recognized branch of surgery is rarely absolute. The surgeon known for colon and rectum work *will* do the occasional appendix or hernia, and may even venture up to the gall bladder with great skill. Nevertheless, the trend is real, probably irreversible, and largely to the patient's benefit. It stands to reason that a surgeon able to collect 50 to 100 cases of a given operation in a year has certain advantages over one doing only three such operations per year. He develops more manipulative skill and detailed anatomical knowledge of the region, but this is probably the least important factor. The real advantage is that he can better assess the place of a given operation in the overall disease process under consideration. He gets to know what factors militate against success, what post-operative pitfalls must be surmounted, what final goals it is realistic to strive for. In short, he achieves perspective and judgement. In fact, a great part of surgical research consists of the painstaking collation and reporting of the fuller knowledge gained in this manner. Specialization also has its disadvantages, and these we will look at in Chapter 12.

## The triumphs and trials of medical therapy

There are two areas in which internal medicine, or more strictly speaking, therapeutics (the branch dealing with administration of drugs for treatment of diseases), has been most successful. The first is in the cure of infections, where the antibiotics have, in every sense of the word, lived up to their popular reputation as wonder drugs. The second is in replacement therapy, to combat diseases due to the lack of some vital substance in the blood. This arises when the organ normally producing that substance has been damaged by disease, when absorption of vital elements of the diet is deranged, or when some process speeds up the normal rate of destruction of the substance concerned. For example, destruction of an endocrine gland, such as the adrenal gland, would once have meant certain death, but now can be effectively treated by giving adrenal hormones. Disease of the stomach lining impairs the normal absorption of vitamin B12 from the diet and causes pernicious anaemia, a severe and previously frequently fatal anaemia. This is adequately managed by periodic vitamin B12 injections. Insulin in diabetes is another example of replacement therapy, though the situation here is complex and the causation of diabetes probably multifactorial.

At the 50th anniversary of the discovery of insulin by Drs. Charles M. Best and Frederick G. Banting, celebrated in 1971, there were eight people still living who had been on insulin for all of those 50 years, instead of dying in childhood or adolescence – living testimony to a signal triumph.

Other major and undoubtedly effective treatments in medicine do not get quite as close to the root of the trouble. For example, drugs of the digitalis group unquestionably strengthen a failing heart. Many people with severe heart disease live longer and more actively and comfortably as a result. Yet, digitalis in no way influences the disease process which is causing that heart to fail. Similarly, blood pressure reducing tablets represent a real breakthrough in therapy of hypertension, and have been proven to prevent heart failure and strokes. However, in a sense they are only symptomatic treatment, as in the majority of cases the reasons why that patient has developed high blood pressure still elude us. Other examples abound, such as anti-depressants and tranquillisers in mental disease, antihistaminics in allergies, dilators of bronchial tubes in asthma, and so forth. The treatment rests on a firm scientific footing and frequently its chemical method of action is well understood. On occasion, it can be as satisfactory from the patient's point of view as a real cure of his illness, because life can go on quite normally and symptoms can be kept at bay by tablets or injections. From a scientific point of view, these treatments are less satisfying than replacement therapy, because the underlying abnormality remains present and, as it is so frequently of unknown cause or nature, it represents a continuing threat.

A third category of drugs belongs to the symptomatic and supportive group. In this unglamorous but important assembly we include pain-relievers, sedatives, laxatives, antacids and so forth. These have a real place, but unfortunately are amongst the most frequently abused. The narcotic drugs of the morphine – heroin group, for example, are unequalled in the relief of pain in advanced cancer, but are also the most dangerous drugs of addiction. I am not competent to write on the drug problem in society, and this would clearly take us far from our central theme. I do believe, however, that I must discuss medical habits with regard to prescribing of drugs. This will lead us to an unfortunate conclusion.

Drugs are useful in the treatment of many diseases. This clear statement is self-evidently true, but needs qualification on two counts. Drugs are useful *if* properly applied and *if* a disease is present. It is my belief that these criteria are met for only a small proportion of the total number of prescriptions written. In general practice, there is frequently a well-established little ritual that is gone through by doctor and patient. The patient presents with symptoms – a fever, a pain, a feeling of nausea – frequently vague, not of long standing, and not severe. Often the illness is trivial and the best treatment consists of reassurance and masterly inactivity. Sometimes the symptoms may be the first manifestation of some real organic disease, and the correct procedure would be, after a thorough medical history is taken and a physical examination has been performed, to order certain specialized diagnostic tests. Alternatively, the physical symptom may be only a superficial manifestation of some domestic or emotional problem, calling for fatherly understanding and patient giving of common sense advice. In none of these hypothetical cases would a prescription of a drug really be called for. Nevertheless, the little ritual demands that the patient should not leave the doctor's consulting rooms empty-handed. The doctor will frequently be overworked and unable to take the time for any of the above lines of action. The patient has often been conditioned to think that a pill or a bottle of medicine is all that is needed to fix him up – a 'tonic', perhaps, or some of those nice capsules with a ring around them that are so expensive (lucky the Government pays!) and therefore must be good. Indeed, if sent on his way without a prescription, the patient may well take a walk up the road to the next doctor!

Perhaps the reader would like to defend the little ritual. After all, what harm do a few tranquillisers or antibiotics do, and if it makes both patient and doctor feel better, does the cost really matter? The answer is clear when one looks at a large population sample. First, all drugs have undesirable side-effects in occasional people, and these can be severe or even fatal. Iatrogenic diseases, that is, diseases caused by the medical profession itself, are by now significant causes of hospital admissions; in particular, adverse reactions to drugs and other idiosyncracies are becoming of increasing concern. Secondly, antibiotic-resistant strains of bacteria appear through injudicious antibiotic usage. Thirdly, the cost factor becomes enormous when applied to a society as a whole. Finally, and most importantly, it is just bad medicine to foster the notion that a pill can make you feel better or can substitute for accurate diagnosis. Pills cannot solve the ordinary day to day worries of life, any more than vitamins or minerals can improve the blood or any other tissue of a healthy person eating a normal diet. The 'tonic' is a mischief, an insult to the intelligence of the patient. The medical profession *can* help people to cope with the stresses of life, but drugs should occupy only a small part of the scene with understanding, compassion, common sense and professional expertise in excluding organic disease all being at the forefront.

Even when organic disease is clearly present, long term usage of drugs should not be undertaken lightly. A decision to commence a regime of blood-pressure reducing tablets may be one that commits the person to treatment for life; cortisone is notoriously difficult to stop once started; the value of long-term anticoagulants in coronary disease or of oral antidiabetic agents in the long-term management of diabetes is still being hotly debated in each case, 20 years after their first introduction. Leading experienced internists deliberate far more deeply before reaching for their prescription pad than is generally realized.

## The difference between aetiology and pathogenesis

Much of the above sounds gloomy and perhaps unfair to the physician. There is some reason for gloom and it relates to the poorly-developed state of our knowledge about the cause of so many diseases. I do not wish to embark on a metaphysical discourse about ultimate causality; in medicine we draw an arbitrary but nevertheless useful distinction between two concepts of disease causation. Aetiology is the word used for basic causes; the aetiology of scurvy is a deficiency of vitamin C in the diet; a virulent streptococcus multiplying on the mucus membranes of the throat is the aetiological agent in scarlet fever. Pathogenesis is the word describing the physiological and biochemical mechanisms by which organs and tissues are damaged in disease. The pathogenesis of a heart attack involves a series of defined steps: a portion of the wall of a coronary vessel becomes roughened and damaged; this leads to narrowing of the aperture of the vessel; this encourages a blood clot to form; that blocks off the vessel and blood stops flowing to the heart muscle; this causes both pain and death of some heart muscle. In other words, the pathogenesis of at least some heart attacks is reasonably well understood. In other cases sudden death mimicking a heart attack may occur in the total absence of autopsy evidence of an actual blockage, and here the presumption is of a disturbance to the normal flow of electrical impulses through the heart, due to poor blood supply. This still leaves open the aetiology, as we do not know enough about why the vessel becomes damaged by the arteriosclerotic process in the first place. The position today about most diseases known to medicine is that pathogenesis is partially or even fully understood but aetiology remains obscure. This fact provides the biggest single justification for a continued massive effort in medical research, and the biggest single reservation about drug treatment of disease.

## Likely contributions of immunology to advances in medical treatment

Immunology, the study of the body's defence system, has become a major specialty in biological and medical science of recent years. This is due not so much to the development of new vaccines, because this has not involved too many new principles, but to a growing realization that immunological processes are important considerations in many diseases. Apart from this, the immune system is a fascinating model of biological engineering. This is not a book of popular immunology, and the reader interested in this aspect is referred to my 'Antibodies and Immunity'. However, I thought it would be useful to summarize briefly those aspects of immunology that seem likely to advance rapidly and to impinge on disease treatment over the next few years. This may represent, in a sense, a microcosm of the wide world of medical research, and may exemplify the extraordinary complexity of the medicine of the future. The four areas that will concern us chiefly are immunization, transplantation, cancer and immune diseases.

## Immunization

There have been some important recent additions to the field of vaccines suitable for human populations, such as measles and german measles (rubella) vaccines, but much remains to be done in the immunization field. A mumps vaccine is near, and consideration is being given to a possible vaccine against the virus responsible for both chicken-pox and shingles. The virus of infectious hepatitis (responsible for attacks of jaundice) remains elusive but progress is being made. The situation for common colds and influenza is a little depressing, because so many different viruses are involved. Immunization is a specific procedure; it is effective against the microorganism used in the vaccine but not against an unrelated one. At least 80 different viruses cause upper respiratory tract infections, and it would not really be practicable to immunize against each of them. This is especially the case as such immunity as is induced by a particular virus infection is of short duration. The 'cure for the common cold' still seems a remote dream.

More research has been devoted to virus vaccines, such as the above, than to new bacterial vaccines. This is because bacteria are usually susceptible to antibiotics whereas viruses are not, and thus bacterial infections can be promptly and effectively treated, making prevention on a mass scale less imperative. However, much more could be done in the immunization field. Vaccines against typhoid fever, whooping cough and cholera could be greatly improved. Vaccines against venereal diseases would, if available, be of great use, especially as antibiotic-resistant forms of V.D. are on the increase. Leprosy can now be effectively treated but not yet prevented by vaccines. It is hard to predict the rate of progress in anti-bacterial immunization, as the level of world-wide effort in this somewhat tedious and less glamourous side of immunology research is much less than that in transplantation or cancer research. I would also welcome a greater research effort in the immunology of protozoal and parasitic infections and other tropical diseases. Much remains to be learnt about malaria, hookworm, sleeping sickness, elephantiasis, schistosomiasis, and many others. It is not clear whether vaccination against any of these would ever be feasible, and many feel that public health measures constitute a sounder line of attack, but an enlarged immunological research effort can be justified on theoretical as well as practical grounds.

## Transplantation

Few advances in medicine have been introduced amidst so much publicity, or have aroused so much controversy, as the field of organ transplantation. The reasons for this are not hard to find. There is something very spectacular and dramatic about replacing an organ that has been destroyed by disease, and whose failing function is threatening the patient's life, with a healthy organ from a living human volunteer or (better still) from a recently deceased person such as a victim of a car accident or a fatal brain haemorrhage. Moreover, when the organ concerned is the human heart, it is little wonder that the public interest is aroused.

Unfortunately, much of the publicity that has filtered down to the average layman has assumed a particularly lurid aspect, and the situation has not been helped by the rather unseemly scurry to get onto the bandwagon which followed the initial few cardiac transplants. Therefore it is important to outline the facts as they are, stressing both the value and the dangers in transplantation procedures, and giving some hints as to the direction that this field is likely to take.

In clinical medicine, the field of organ transplantation is usually thought of in terms of the saving of relatively young lives. Most deaths in people over say 65 or 70 years are due to diseases that are widely diffused through the body. Hardening of the arteries (arterio-sclerosis) and cancer are the two most common, but there are many other examples. In younger people, multiple organ diseases are also common, but there is still a large group of serious disorders where essentially only one organ has gone wrong. The commonest cause of death in middle aged men, for example, is a heart attack. This is due to the occlusion of a blood vessel bringing oxygen to the heart muscle. Sometimes, the disease in the blood vessel which leaves the blockage is widespread through the body, but often it is practically confined to the small arteries supplying the heart. The whole person dies because of malfunction of one working part. There are other serious, common disorders which do not kill quickly but impair health and shorten life. Among these is diabetes, which is due to poor function of certain cells in the pancreas. A reasonably common cause of death in younger life is chronic kidney disease. This may be the end result of repeated infections, or due to the progress of various types of autoimmune disorders. Primarily, it is to all those disorders due to the failure of a particular organ that the field of transplantation is most relevant. The concept involves substitution of a good organ for the one destroyed by disease. If it were possible to use all the healthy organs of all people who die from whatever cause to replace effectively the diseased organs of sick people, the savings in human life and suffering would be incalculable. We are a very long way from that goal, but still closer to it than anyone would have dreamed possible as recently as a decade ago.

## Early experiences in human organ transplantation

The tissue that was first extensively used in transplantation was skin. During World War II, much experimentation went on about the use of skin grafts, from both cadavers and volunteers, to cover large areas in victims suffering from burns. It was noticed that this physiological method of treating burns did indeed provide a very satisfactory first-aid dressing, helpful in the prevention of excessive fluid loss and in reducing infection. However, the skin never 'took' permanently. Unlike skin taken from a healthy portion of the burnt patient's body, which healed and became fully integrated into its new locality, the skin transplanted from another individual, within a very few weeks, died and was sloughed off. We owe to the Scottish plastic surgeon Thomas Gibson and the British biologist Sir Peter Medawar the realization that this rejection process represented an immune response on the part of the lymphocytes of the burnt patient.

The techniques for skin transplantation were well established, as grafting of skin from one area of the body to another is part of the daily stock in trade of the plastic surgeon. However, with the kidney it was another matter. A complex organ such as the kidney is not as tough as skin. It will only survive in a transplantation situation if an adequate blood supply is established within an hour or so of its removal from the donor. This statement is subject to the reservation that techniques of organ preservation, of a rather complex and technical nature, and involving perfusion of the kidney with blood-like fluids, are making rapid strides. Therefore, clearly kidney transplantation could not be entertained until surgical techniques had been developed to enable the suturing of very fine vessels involving in this case the artery and vein of the kidney and also the tube which leads urine from the kidney to the bladder, called the ureter. We owe much to an intrepid team of surgeons in Boston who pioneered the technique of kidney transplantation. Unfortunately, their early work ran into trouble, again because of host immunological defences, but it did show that kidney transplantation was technically feasible, and that the transplanted kidney functioned remarkably well until the processes of immunological rejection got under way.

The only exception to the rule of immune rejection is the case of identical twins. Here we are dealing with two individuals derived from a single fertilized ovum, and therefore having exactly the same complement of genetic material. Identical twins are alike in their blood groups and also in the genes (called histocompatibility genes) responsible for determining the chemical nature of the cell surface, and so a transplanted kidney will be identical in its chemistry to the kidney of the recipient. Thus, the cellular immune attack does not occur, and if the transplant has been satisfactorily performed from a surgical viewpoint, it will be a long-range success. The only danger is that the kidney disease which initially attacked the patient's own kidney may, some years later, recur in the transplanted kidney; and we are getting much better at preventing this from happening.

## Medical aids to transplantation

We now have a variety of ways of minimizing the onslaught of the immune system against the transplanted organ. These fall under four chief headings. First, there are genetic matching techniques which can minimize the chemical disparity between donor and host, and thus result in less vigorous lymphocyte invasion. Secondly, we have drugs that slow down the division rate of aggressive lymphocytes and damp down the cellular immune attack. Thirdly, we can combine these with other drugs, chiefly of the cortisone group, which lessen the inflammatory damage resulting from the lymphocyte's onslaught on its target tissue. Fourthly, we employ a specific lymphocyte poison called antilymphocyte serum. This is, in fact, an antibody made by injecting horses or goats with human lymphocytes. The animal is bled, the antibody is suitably purified, and when the antibody is injected into the transplant recipient, the lymphocytes anxious to destroy the organ graft are instead themselves destroyed.

Unfortunately, these various immunosuppressive measures weaken the patient's own capacity to ward off infections, and this is a serious problem, particularly in the early stages after operation, when the immune attack on the graft is at its height, and the doses of immunosuppressives at their maximum. Intensive research is in progress to find better aids to transplant survival.

## Clinical results of transplantation for the various organs

The organ that has been transplanted far more frequently than any other is the kidney. In fact, the world organ transplant registry, run jointly by the American College of Surgeons and National Institutes of Health, recorded that 16,691 kidney transplants had been reported between 1951 and 1974, and it is estimated that in 1974 over 4,000 transplants will be performed by over 200 surgical teams around the world. In contrast, by March, 1, 1974, only 232 heart transplants had been performed by a total of 63 surgical teams, and of these only 33 were alive with functioning grafts. The longest of these has been in place for 5.5 years. There have been 39 liver, 21 lung and 12 pancreas transplants reported. The success of renal transplantation has been very encouraging. Results are near perfect for identical twins and the best centres are obtaining satisfactory results in about 80% of living volunteer transplants and about 60% in cadaveric transplants. The longest living transplant recipient has had the graft in place for 18 years. One further gains the impression that results are improving all the time, as groups build up greater experience. The reason that the kidney leads the field so clearly is not that there is something rather special about the histocompatibility antigens of kidney. Rather, it arises from a number of circumstances. First of all, renal transplantation is technically much easier for the surgeon than the transplantation of organs such as the liver or the lung. Secondly, and much more importantly, the renal transplant patient can be got into very satisfactory preoperative condition by the use of the artificial kidney. This is a machine which removes waste matter from the blood that is shunted through it from the patient's circulation. In fact, if the transplant is a failure, the patient can go back onto the artificial kidney two or three times per week and await his chance of a further transplantation. However, formidable problems of logistics and finance limit the degree to which such chronic haemodialysis programmes can be maintained.

In general, the results of heart transplantation so far have been rather disappointing, but there is a handful of quite notable exceptions of patients who live for over a year with another heart. Although the total world figures show only 20% of patients living for 12 months and 11% living for 3 years, certain of the most experienced groups have obtained better results than this. For example, the Stanford University group under Dr. Norman Shumway reports 30% surviving to two years. Factors which one might cite as creating special difficulties in heart transplantation include the very poor condition of patients when they present for the operation (obviously no one would contemplate replacing a person's heart unless the patient were on the very brink of death) and the absence of any support device such as the artificial kidney to help the patient over rough spots. Kidney patients can afford to have a poorly functioning organ for days or even weeks; if a heart transplant patient has a rejection crisis, it is a much more serious matter. The worst problem, however, relates to the development in the heart transplant recipients of a very severe vascular disease in the blood vessels going to the heart muscle itself. It appears that it is the lining of the blood vessels that bear the brunt of the immunological attack, and the severe vessel wall disease appears in transplant recipients despite best efforts at immunosuppression. This immunological coronary vessel disease is curiously like the spontaneous coronary artery disease which causes heart attacks. This has even led researchers to wonder whether some forms of spontaneous coronary artery disease might be immunological in origin.

Liver transplantation, though extraordinarily difficult technically, is making steady progress in three or four selected centres. Obviously, as for heart, one can think only of cadaver donors. A liver transplantation is a much more difficult operation than a heart transplantation, as the post operative technical surgical complications which ensue are, unfortunately, rather frequent and serious. Again, there is only a handful of long term successes to report in this field to date, but progress is being made.

Lung transplantation in the main has been extremely disappointing in the experimental animal, and, probably for this reason, relatively little work has been done in man. One or two apparently successful lung transplants have been reported. However, the lung is an organ with an extremely rich capillary blood supply, and as the lining of blood vessels is such a vulnerable target for immunological attack, the lung would seem to be an especially difficult organ to transplant from the immunological viewpoint. It seems likely that this operation will only become feasible when better methods of immunological control are available than today.

Most diabetics are treated adequately by injections of insulin, but some go on to develop severe kidney complications. There have been a series of such cases treated with combined transplantation of pancreas and kidney. Again we are dealing with a heroic surgical exercise, and so far survival has been limited to a few months in most cases. Two patients surviving for almost two years have been reported. Similarly depressing comments can be made about the few attempts to transplant large segments of intestine.

As the non-renal field will probably look somewhat bleak to the reader, let us end on a more cheerful note. There are many less dramatic transplantation procedures that have a high success rate. The best known is the cornea of the eye, which normally has no blood supply and is relatively inaccessible to attacking lymphocytes. Also, many materials are of low inherent antigenicity, particularly after the cells in them have been destroyed by some preservative. These include tissues such as cartilage, tendons, bone chips, sheets of fascia and walls of large blood vessels such as the aorta (always provided the vulnerable inner lining is not present). Transplants of tissues such as these form an important part of eye surgery, plastic and reconstructive surgery, and orthopaedic surgery. However, in many cases, components constructed from metal or plastics have proven so successful in reconstructive surgery that the need for transplantation is lessening.

The reason for maintaining a certain guarded optimism about transplantation of major organs other than the kidney is that the methods of immunological control, and indeed the level of understanding of the problems involved, are increasing steadily.

## Future of transplantation

I believe the transplantation field is here to stay, but how far it will revolutionize the fabric of medicine remains to be seen. It is not unreasonable to hope that our power to control the immune attack will continue to increase, but it may not become absolute, or at least not in the next 10 to 15 years. This would mean that many transplants would continue to live in an uneasy kind of truce with their hosts. Availability of donor organs is obviously another big problem area, as the transplant barrier will be much harder to overcome for organs from chimpanzees or other primates. Artificial organs may well find a place and may even come to challenge transplants one day. An even rosier hope is that better medical treatment and diagnosis at earlier stages will prevent the extensive destruction of organs that now makes transplantation seem so frequently desirable.

## The immune system and cancer

Cancer is widely regarded as one of the three most challenging problems left for medical science to tackle. The other two are heart and arterial diseases, and mental disease. Many people have a morbid fear of cancer, a fear which is not helped by the widespread ignorance about the central facts. Cancer is indeed a killer – it ranks second only to heart and arterial diseases in mortality statistics for most Western communities. In fact, about one person in five will eventually die of cancer. It is disturbing to find how often quite intelligent and educated people will stop you in the street and ask 'Have you a ray of hope in the cancer field yet? How long will it be till we have a cure?' Of course the fact is that some cancers can be prevented and many can already be cured. Our knowledge of the cancer process and our ability to prolong lives is increasing constantly. As cancer undoubtedly represents a wide spectrum of different diseases, it is unlikely that a sudden breakthrough or panacea cure will suddenly emerge, and certainly no responsible investigator would claim that an immunological approach will soon bring all the answers. However, numerous useful links between immunology and cancer research are developing, and the exploration is proving helpful to both disciplines. Therefore, we shall examine what impact immunology has had on cancer research so far.

What is cancer? It is a form of overgrowth of tissue that we term a malignant tumour. Tumours or neoplasms are the names that we give to any growth of tissue that is beyond the limits of health or normalcy. A gardener will get callouses on his hands and a weightlifter will find certain muscles grow in size. These are normal responses of body cells to extensive usage. Tumours are growths which fall outside this range. They can be broadly divided into benign or malignant tumours.

Benign tumours, as the name implies, grow relatively slowly. They do not grossly invade the surrounding tissues or diffuse widely through the body. A good example of a benign tumour is an ordinary mole; another, the round, fatty lumps that quite a few people have on their backs or elsewhere, which are called lipomas. If a benign tumour is externally situated, it has at worst a cosmetically harmful effect. However, benign tumours in internal organs can be quite serious and even fatal. For example, a benign tumour in the brain can grow very slowly, causing no symptoms at all until it begins to press on vital nerve centres. If surgery is then undertaken, a complete cure can result, but if the case is left untreated, the patient may eventually die.

A malignant tumour is characterized by more rapid growth, invasion of surrounding tissue and tendency to spread through the lymphocytes or via the bloodstream to give satellite areas of tumour growth, usually called metastases or secondaries, in organs remote from the original tumour site. Unfortunately, malignant tumours are quite common in both sexes, particularly with advancing age. The commonest internal cancers are those of the lungs, large intestine, stomach, and, in the appropriate sex, breast, uterus and prostate. If a cancer is treated by surgery (or in certain cases by high doses of irradiation) before spread from the original growth site has occurred, then a total cure will usually result. If spread is confined to the local draining lymph nodes a careful dissection of these and total removal can succeed in achieving a cure, but this is less common. If widespread metastases are present, total cure is highly unlikely but a variety of treatments exist which can give the patient years of extra useful life free of pain. Even in this area, the prospects are not quite as gloomy as they were.

It is rather doubtful whether it is proper to refer to cancer as a single disease entity. In all probability, cancer is a blanket term which describes a number of totally different and possibly causally unrelated conditions. In the last century an enormous amount of observational knowledge has been collected about human cancer. We can give quite elaborate and detailed descriptions of the microscopic appearance and growth behaviour of cancers of each organ. We have many helpful diagnostic tests to allow early detection. We can give accurate statistical estimates of the likely responses of the different forms of cancer to treatment. In a few instances such as lung cancer, or skin cancers of white Australians living in the northern states, we can describe the most probable causative factor – cigarette smoking, on the one hand, and excessive exposure of fair-skinned people to the sun, on the other. All work on human cancer is subject to the constraint that deliberate experimentation on man is not possible, except in the context of therapeutic trial. Obviously, one cannot perform experiments designed to test the cancer-inducing potential or carcinogenicity of chemicals, irritants or viruses by applying them directly to human populations. Because of this, we have only primitive insight into the origins, causes, and predisposing factors in the various malignancies. For this reason, many researchers in the cancer field have devoted their lives to a study of cancer in experimental animals, predominantly mice. This is motivated by the hope that a thorough understanding of the causes and effects of cancer in the mouse will illuminate the darker aspects of our knowledge of cancer in man. Virtually all our knowledge of the immunology of cancer comes from work on inbred mice, and we have already realized that humans are far from being a genetically uniform population. It may therefore be worthwhile to issue a chastening reminder that the direct relevance of much recent advance in cancer immunology to human malignancies remains to be proven.

## Theories on the causes of cancer

There are basically three major theories on the way that cancer arises, and it is important to realize at once that these are not mutually exclusive. First, it is known that certain chemicals can lead to cancerous changes in tissues, particularly if these are applied in a repeated fashion over long periods. Good experimental examples are the application of coal tar to the skin (where the carcinogenic hydrocarbons lead to skin cancers) or the ingestion of certain dyes which predictably lead to the development of liver cancer. It is clear that lung cancer in man belongs to this group of chemically-induced malignancies. Bladder cancers frequent in workers in certain dye factories provide another example, as did the old fashioned carcinoma of the scrotum amongst chimney sweeps. In this latter example, and in many laboratory counterparts, mechanical irritation probably played a helping role in cancer induction. It is known, also, that radiation such as strong ultraviolet rays from sunlight or ionizing radiation such as from nuclear fall-out or an X-ray machine, may heighten the incidence of certain cancers. The linking factor between chemical carcinogenesis and radiation – induced carcinogenesis is that both probably act by damaging the DNA molecules of the cell nucleus. Elaborate DNA repair mechanisms exist, but if these fail, an altered or 'mutant' cell with changed growth characteristics may result.

The second major inductive force in cancer is virus infection. In experimental animals, it is clear that certain viruses can induce a variety of tumours, the case perhaps being best established for leukaemia. However, we are by no means dealing with an ordinary infectious event as is the case for influenza or measles. In fact, most cancer viruses thought to be responsible for animal cancer are transmitted not by direct contact or air borne infection, but 'vertically' from parent to offspring. In the case of many cancer viruses, infection is very widely spread through the body, even though only certain organs actually develop tumours. Therefore a pregnant mouse may pass the virus to its embryos at a very early stage of its development. In many cases, the actual development of cancer depends upon subtle interaction between the virus and the genetic constitution of the infected animal. Thus, leukaemia can be produced in one strain of mice but not in another. The degree of genetic involvement is far greater than is the case for most normal infections. All of this adds up to the fact that virus infection may be only one of several factors leading to the eventual malignant process.

In the human, we cannot state with certainty whether any cancer is caused by a virus. Very active work on the isolation of a possible leukaemia virus is going on, but it would be fair to say that the work so far has been less conclusive than that in experimental animals. There are two other malignancies in which strong hints of a viral association are present. The first is a tumour of the jaw occurring chiefly in Africans, and termed Burkitt's lymphoma; and the second is a cancer occurring in the tissue at the back of the nose and throat, chiefly in Chinese. In both cases, it is suspected that a virus similar to the agent which causes glandular fever is involved. Viruses of the same general group have also been claimed to be implicated in cancer of the uterine cervix and in Hodgkin's disease, though this remains highly controversial. Of course, the key puzzle is that vastly greater numbers of people become infected with the glandular fever virus than ever develop these relatively rare cancers. This is just another illustration of the confused state of cancer virology, and of the probably dominant importance of genetic considerations.

The third theory of cancer origin relates to the possibility that the cancer cell really represents a reversion to an embryonic pattern of cell division. It is a characteristic of embryonic cells to create an ever-enlarging cell population. The evidence for the embryonic reversion idea comes from immunology, as we shall see below. Two key examples of where embryonic reversion has been claimed for human cancers are cancer of the liver and cancer of the colon.

From a human point of view, the key thing to remember about cancer-promoting influences, be these viruses, chemicals, irritants or virtually unknown factors, is that not all people are at equal risk. It is sheer commonsense to avoid such obvious promoting factors as cigarette smoking, but there are still so many unknowns, particularly in relation to the importance of host genetic factors, that there is little virtue in brooding over possibilities.

## Tumour-specific antigens

The key contribution that immunology has made so far to the cancer field is the realization that cancer cells are immunologically different from the normal cells of the patient or animal bearing the cancer. In other words, there are chemical groupings on the surface of a cancer cell that are sufficiently different from the normal components of membranes of normal cells for that difference to be recognized immunologically. It is possible to prepare antibodies against these so-called tumour-specific antigens. Most of the antigens concerned are rather weak ones, and so the amount of antibody against tumour-specific antigens made by an animal injected with cancer cells is small. Various specialized techniques have to be used to prepare tumour-specific antibodies. Once again, it appears that identifiable tumour-specific antigens fall into three groups: virally induced; chemically-induced; and embryonic. However, there are some important differences between the three varieties. In the case of virally-induced tumour-specific antigens, a given cancer virus will cause the appearance of the same antigen in each of twenty mice having the relevant cancer. In the case of chemically-induced malignancies, the same chemical can be used to cause cancer in twenty mice, but the detailed chemical properties of the tumour-specific antigen will be different in each of the twenty. This is because it is believed that the chemical really promotes the emergence of certain somatic mutations amongst cells, and as mutations are a random process, there is no reason why the mutation should take exactly the same form in the twenty cases. Thirdly, the embryonic type tumour-specific antigen is different from the normal adult pattern of cells, but there is similarity to antigens present on the surface of perfectly normal embryo cells.

There are practical consequences flowing from these differences in tumour-specific antigens. If one were ever to contemplate using a tumour cell as a kind of vaccine for cancer treatment, it is clear that for those cancers that are of a virally induced nature, the cancer of person A would serve as a sort of universal vaccine, having antigens on its surface identical to that of patients B, C, D and E, provided always that we are dealing with the identical cancer. On the other hand, for chemically induced malignancies there is something unique about the tumour-specific antigens of patient A, and the only potential source for a vaccine would be the cancer cells of the actual patient himself. In the case of embryonic tumour-specific antigens, the situation would be similar to that pertaining in virally induced cancers. Different patients with the same form of cancer would exhibit the same embryonic antigen.

## Possibilities of immunotherapy in cancer

At this stage, many readers will be wondering about the question of whether all of this work on tumour-specific antigens has any practical consequences. The answer is that while no thoroughly evaluated immunotherapeutic manoeuvre has yet gained full acceptance in the medical literature for any form of cancer, much human clinical trial work is proceeding, and it seems highly likely that, within five years at least, some forms of cancer will be being treated routinely by immunotherapy.

If cancer cells are antigenically different from normal cells, why does the body's immune system not mount an attack on the cancer rather similar to the attack that is mounted on a foreign organ transplant? There are three answers to this question. The first is that almost certainly many cancers are defeated by the vigilance of the immune system before they ever arise – nipped in the bud, as it were. In fact many authorities believe that the key reason why the cellular immune system really evolved is as a kind of surveillance mechanism against cancer. The second point is that tumour-specific antigens are only slightly different from the normal components of host cell membranes, and thus they are weak antigens. The immune response against them is feeble, and there may be instances where the unaided immune system of the patient cannot win out against the intense proliferative drive of the abnormal cancer cell. In this case we have a war waged between cancer and host defences, but being won by the cancer. The third explanation is more subtle, and involves a new concept which is too technical to explain in detail. It turns out that there are two kinds of lymphocytes, one of which, called the T lymphocyte, is good at fighting the cancer. The other type, the B lymphocyte, can actually help the cancer to grow. This paradoxical activity of the B lymphocyte is termed tumour enhancement or immunological enhancement.

What might the goals of an immunological approach to cancer actually be? First and foremost, it is hoped that all of these branches of research will give us a fuller insight into the nature of the cancer process. In many respects it is pointless to speculate much further than this, particularly as the whole field is moving so rapidly at the present time. Amongst the readily forseeable goals, however, are the following:

1. Identification of tumour-specific antigens, or antibodies against tumour-specific antigens, may be a considerable help in the early and correct diagnosis of cancer, particularly because of the known sensitivity of immunological methods.

2. It might be possible to devise ways of immunizing patients with cancer against their own tumour-specific antigens present on the cancer cells, in such a way as to activate selectively the T lymphocyte system, thus providing a family of killer cells and avoiding the problem of immunological enhancement.

3. It may be possible to chemically couple anticancer drugs or radioactive isotopes to anti-tumour antibodies, thus providing a kind of golden bullet that brings the destructive agent selectively to the site of the cancer.

4. In certain selected cases, it may be possible to identify cancer-promoting viruses and to vaccinate whole communities against these,

although at the present time this goal seems further in the distance than some of the other ones.

## Conventional treatment of cancer

Quite apart from these speculative matters just discussed, it must not be forgotten that there are a number of very effective methods of treating cancer available already in clinical medicine. Chief amongst these are surgery, radiation with deep X-rays or some other form of ionizing radiation, and the use of a variety of drugs which influence the rate of cell division, this last area being termed chemotherapy. There is thus no reason for the cancer patient to despair. Apart from the hope generated through immunology research, it is wise to stress that prevention through the avoidance of known carcinogenic influences and early diagnosis, together with early treatment, represent the corner-stones of any sensible approach to cancer.

## Immunological diseases

Another area that has spurred on the present immunology research explosion is that of immunological diseases. It is now recognized that the pathogenesis of many diseases that had previously been poorly understood is due to immune responses gone wrong. First, we have the so-called autoimmune diseases. These result when the lymphocytes turn traitors, and mount an immune attack on some bodily tissue, such as the liver, kidney or a component of blood. It is believed that many chronic disorders, including rheumatoid arthritis, pernicious anaemia, the thyroid diseases and a whole range of other conditions, are of autoimmune nature. The second group of immunological disorders is one in which antibodies are formed against some microorganism that enters the body, and in which the resulting neutralization of bacterial products forms a so-called antigen-antibody complex, which can cause irritation in the body in a variety of ways. Acute nephritis is an example of 'immune complex' disease. Thirdly, a special type of antibody can be formed against particulate bits of foreign matter such as grass pollens, household dust, feathers and so forth. In some patients, this antibody fixes onto cells in the lining of the respiratory tract. When next the antigen or 'allergen' comes along, the union of antigen and antibody on cell surfaces can cause the release of powerful stored chemicals, resulting in manifestations such as hay fever or asthma. This third group constitutes the allergic diseases.

Research into these and other miscellaneous immune diseases constitutes the relatively new specialty of immunopathology. This has as its aim the discovery of better treatments based on deeper understanding of aetiology and pathogenesis. Recent progress towards cures has not been spectacular and it is difficult to be too optimistic about this field in the short to medium term. Nevertheless, the progressive unravelling of the chemical steps involved should help the development of better drugs eventually.

## Immunological engineering

There is a 'brave new world' branch of transplantation which involves immunology in a special way and which deserves a brief comment. It is the transplantation into a person of the immune system itself! Mostly when organ transplantation is considered, one thinks of a single organ such as the kidney, liver, lung or heart. The immune system, on the other hand, is widely deployed round the body rather than concentrated in a single organ. Thus thymus, bone marrow, spleen, lymph nodes and other organized collections of lymphatic tissue, together with circulating cells in the blood and lymph, constitute a dynamic whole. There are certain diseases in which one or more types of lymphocytes are congenitally absent from this pool. Some quirk of development has led to a defect in the differentiation of cells. This leaves the child with a crippled or absent immune defence system.

Grafts of thymus or bone marrow from a volunteer or cadaver may appear to be the answer. However, these cells are themselves immunologically active. This time it is *not* a question of the host lymphocytes killing the graft, as the host is an immunological cripple. Rather, the donor lymphocytes constituting the graft recognize the foreignness of their new home and begin to mount an immune attack on the host. Such a 'graft versus host' reaction can be quite violent, and can kill the child.

Immunological engineering can come in at this point. Techniques are now available not only for better matching of donor and host or for drug control of the graft versus host reaction, but also for actual separation of different kinds of cells in the graft. For example, one can separate off the 'stem' cells capable of re-equipping the host lymphoid system from the 'killer' cells is also relevant to treatment of some forms of anaemia and leukaemia. The word immunological engineering has been coined because the sequence of science-based steps leading to a successful procedure is quite complex and multi-component, in contrast to the frequently rather empiric drug treatments that form the basis of most of clinical medicine. How far we can go in this process of greater complexity in medical treatment will depend largely on community decisions relating to the level of funds available for health and for hospitals in particular. We have looked at one area of medicine only, but the pattern is exactly the same for many other fields, and the costs of this new form of scientific hospital medicine are escalating in an alarming manner. As for so many problems of modern society, solutions will be partial and compromises inevitable.

*Further reading*

Burnet, F. M. *Immunological Surveillance,* Pergamon Press, Oxford (1970).
Nossal, G. J. V. *Antibodies and Immunity,* Penguin Books, (1971).
Wolstenholme, G. W. ed., *Man and his Future,* Ciba Foundation. J. and A. Churchill Ltd., London (1963).

# 10

# Medical research and the evolution of mankind

'*Man as a scientist can provide practical control of phenomena. It is for man as man to control that control*'. Julian Huxley

Once in recent history, the dramatic suddenness with which fundamental scientific discoveries led to practical applications of overwhelming importance for mankind caught both scientists and society by surprise. The agony of the atomic scientists before and after Hiroshima was just as real as the anxiety and bewilderment of the rest of the world. Due to the war-time pressures of and the conviction mistaken as it turned out, that Hitler was on the track of an A-bomb, circumstances were not favourable for a dispassionate analysis of the social implications of nuclear research. Will it happen again? Biology has undergone a revolution just as profound in its own way as the atomic revolution in physics that occurred in the early 1900's. What implications will this have for mankind's evolution, and what preparations should we be making to avoid unpleasant surprises?

As Huxley has indicated, the scientist does not stand alone with answers to this question. He will extend his powers over both laboratory and real life situations, but the pace and penetration of the application of new scientific knowledge remains dependent on a dynamic symbiosis between science and society.

So far in this book, we have tended to confine our attention to conventional medical and scientific research, and to the way this affects individual health in Western communities. In this chapter, we must explore the wider and longer-range consequences of modern advances in biology for the species as a whole. We must endeavour to steer a course between the irresponsible alarmism of those who warn that 'people from cuttings are just around the corner', and the complacency of those who claim that the biologists' toys and dreams will never leave the test tube or impinge on real life. What are the facts?

Darwin's *Origin of Species* was published in 1859, and, though his ideas on evolution had been widely discussed in scientific circles before that time, we should probably take 1859 as the year of birth of modern biology. Darwin (and independently Wallace) reached two conclusions. First, the survival and proliferation of a living species depend on a cruel struggle between it and its environment; as the environment (climate, sources of food, number and strength of predators) changes, so the chances for survival become better or worse. Those individuals in the species best fitted to cope with a changed environment are the ones which survive and reproduce. Secondly, the basis of evolution is random variation amongst individuals, rather than the passing on of acquired characteristics from generation to generation. In other words, the fitness to survive is not something that can be transmitted through individual striving and effort. Such exercise of will and spirit might help an individual to survive, but nothing learnt in the struggle can be passed on; stretch its neck as it might, the giraffe could not help its progeny to a longer neck. Mendel was able to add an important perspective in uncovering some of the rules of genetics, the laws that govern the way in which hereditary characteristics are passed on. The fundamental validity of Darwinian natural selection as the basis of evolution of species is now no longer questioned, and even before the era of molecular biology, much information about the nature of the gene and the basis and frequency of mutations was available.

What molecular biology has achieved is to give defined chemical shape and precision to the science of genetics. Avery and Griffiths established that the genetic material in the cell nucleus was a substance known as desoxyribonucleic acid or DNA; Watson and Crick worked out the detailed structure of DNA; and Monod and Jacob laid the foundations of our understanding of the regulatory principles governing gene activation. Literally thousands of scientists have followed on and given us a very satisfying insight into the machinery of simple living organisms such as viruses and bacteria. Of course, the information is not complete, but the outlines of nature's plans are clear. We know that DNA encodes the instructions for the synthesis of the cell's workhorse molecules, the proteins. We know the code in detail: a sequence of three letters out of DNA's four letter alphabet (thus giving $4 \times 4 \times 4$ or 64 possible code words) codes for a single building block of protein. As there are only twenty different kinds of protein building blocks or amino acids, there is information to spare, and many amino acids can be called up by several different triplets of nucleic acid. The genetic information stored in DNA is transcribed into a kind of intermediary template called messenger RNA before being used in actual protein synthesis. The detailed building-block sequence of many proteins and some messenger RNA molecules is now known and a number of proteins have been made in the test tube from their individual building blocks. As a bacterial cell makes some three thousand different proteins, it will be some time yet before its inner workings are completely known.

Larger organisms such as mammals are obviously much more complex still. However, it has been determined that the triplet code is universal – all living organisms from the humblest to the proudest, including microbes, plants, birds and animals, use the same basic mechanisms for synthesis of proteins and maintenance of hereditary stability. The starting point for Darwinian evolution is mutation, or an occasional copying error in DNA duplication. When a cell divides, it duplicates its DNA, and if a copying error ensues, an incorrect nucleotide building block is inserted. When the time comes for that gene to be activated, the particular triplet in which the incorrect building block occurs will usually now code for a different amino acid, and the protein eventually built will accordingly have a slightly different shape and properties. In the majority of cases, the copying error, will result in poorer function as the protein structure concerned is itself the product of the long evolutionary process and thus its exquisite design not lightly tampered with. Occasionally it will happen that the mutant protein is functionally more effective than the previous one in the particular environment in which the cell finds itself. Then the cell possessing the mutation will have a survival advantage over its neighbours.

When a mutation happens in any cell of a higher organism other than the germ cells (the ancestor cells of eggs and sperms), the consequences, be they good or evil, are confined to that particular individual. This kind of mutation we term a somatic mutation, and while somatic mutations may be of importance in cancer and other diseases, by definition they cannot influence the progeny of the individual. However, when a mutation happens in a germ cell, the results are felt by the offspring, and he may, through the chance of mutation, be better fitted to survive in a particular environment. Sexual reproduction, in which genetic characteristics of two different individuals are randomly mixed up and reassorted in the progeny, greatly increases the pre-determined diversity on which natural selection can act.

From the viewpoint of this book, the most important question is whether this new knowledge of the chemistry and regulation of heredity has any practical significance. This is a contentious issue, and will occupy us for much of this chapter.

## Problems in human evolution

In the human species, and particularly Western communities over the last two hundred years, the rules of the evolutionary game have changed.

Darwinian survival of the fittest is a cruel process, and civilized man has softened its impact on his own development. Thus, we look after the sick, the weak, the mentally retarded and many other individuals who, in a survival test in animal kingdom terms, would succumb to a predator or at least not succeed in winning a mate. In particular, medical science is allowing people with previously fatal genetically-determined abnormalities, such as diabetes or haemophilia, to survive to the age of marriage, and to have children. This is not to say that evolutionary forces are not at work in the human. Not everyone gets married, and not all married couples have an equal number of children. Many factors no doubt determine the 'breeding habits' of humans, most of which defy detailed analysis. The point is that the determining issues are no longer related to simple natural imperatives such as capacity to hunt and kill, ability to survive extremes of temperature, skill in coping with rival species, and so forth. The patterns of human reproduction are now largely dictated by social and cultural forces. Another and perhaps more frightening way of saying the same thing is to declare that the directions of man's evolution are now largely in his own hands – a situation without precedent in nature. To this must be added the fact that cultural patterns are passed on from generation to generation through the processes of tradition and learning, and these may be every bit as important as genetic mechanisms, particularly in the relatively short term. Thus, in more ways than one, man's future is in his own hands.

## Positive and negative eugenics

Eugenics is the science which deals with attempts at improving the human species through selective breeding. There are really two types of eugenics which we can describe as positive and negative. Positive eugenics aims at encouraging a society to produce more children from those parents that have characteristics deemed to be desirable. Though various eminent people including Nobel Laureates have been strong advocates of positive eugenics, it has never really got off the ground, and for what I consider to be very good reasons. First, how can we agree on what human traits are desirable? To Adolf Hitler, the various characteristics of so-called pure Aryan Germans were desirable; the emphasis which he placed on conventional intelligence can be gauged by his treatment of the Jews. Even if we leave monstrosities of genocide aside, there would be wide disagreement amongst sensitive and humanistically inclined people about the relative importance of, for example, intelligence, energy and drive, or physical strength and fitness. What eugenicist would set himself up as a judge between a doctor, a film star, a champion golfer or a trade union leader in terms of being worthy of having progeny? Secondly, even if there were a prospect of reaching consensus on who should be a parent, it would be an affront to human dignity and individual freedom to legislate in an appropriate manner. Thirdly, most of the human traits that seem desirable are not simple genetic dominants or recessives, but of multicomponent nature and of poorly-understood genetic origin.

Negative eugenics seems to me a more realistic goal at which to aim. This is an attempt to minimize the transmission into future generations of genetic traits that are clearly negative or harmful. Many defects and diseases are of hereditary nature, and some gloomy predictions have been made about the accumulation of these in societies with progressively more elaborate medical care systems. My standpoint on this issue is quite clear. I believe that it would be proper for society to use educational pressure to urge people with known genetic defects to forsake having children or to severely restrict the number of their children. I do not believe that I would care to live in a society where this pressure turned into force. Legislation for compulsory sterilization on the basis of some defect that is not in any way a person's fault offends my deep-seated and perhaps not very scientifically conceived sense of human value. Educational standards in Western communities have risen remarkably in two hundred years, and there is no reason to believe that this trend will not continue at an equal pace over the next two hundred. As enlightenment about man's genetic and biological nature spreads, so issues concerning procreation will come more fully into the arena of public cognisance and debate. There has already been a change in the way that educated people view family numbers. The need for restraint at the personal level has come into much clearer focus. A similar trend for self-assessment in terms of possession of negative genes will take much longer but would require only a logical extension of the same social forces.

## Markers for genetic defects

From a technical viewpoint, human genetics is making rapid progress. To understand this, we must go back to a consideration of the DNA-RNA-protein relationship. When there is a mutation (copying error) in DNA, the end result is an altered protein. This statement must be somewhat qualified for higher animals, because in these there are two full sets of chromosomes, or strings of genes; one inherited from the father and one from the mother. In some cases, both genes of a pair are expressed but in others one gene of the pair dominates and the other is not overtly expressed. Genes of this type are referred to as 'recessive' genes. The existence of recessive genes gives scientific validation to the well-known dangers of inbreeding. If a person has a bad recessive gene, this may be partially or totally masked by the presence of the paired, good dominant gene. What happens when the person marries a partner who also carries one good and one bad gene for that particular trait? Let us abbreviate the good, dominant gene as G, and the bad, recessive gene as B. We can then say that the genotype of each parent for that particular trait is GB. However, as the good gene dominates in the example chosen, the actual biochemistry of the person's cells is G. Technically, we say that the person expresses the *phenotype* G, or is phenotypically G for that characteristic. Now, when a father of genotype GB (phenotypically G and thus perfectly healthy) marries a mother of genotype GB (therefore also healthy) there is a random reassortment of the genes in the progeny according to the rules worked out by Mendel. Statistically, one in four offspring will be genotype GG; one in four BB; and two in four GB. Phenotypically, three in four will be G (healthy) but one in four B, i.e. sick with whatever disease or defect may be occasioned by the bad gene. We refer to individuals of genotype GB as *carriers* of the particular defective trait.

There are some genetic diseases where the defective gene trait is dominant rather than recessive. Here the individual genotypically GB would be phenotypically B. Interestingly enough, this situation presents less of a problem as there is an inherent tendency (if the resulting disease is severe) for the patients to realize the legacy they are bestowing on their children, and to avoid procreating. Also, they may die before reaching marriageable age. In other words, such diseases remain rare in the community, except if they occur in very small, highly inbred population groups. Unfortunately, there are many diseases, such as diabetes and autoimmune diseases, where there is a certain degree of genetic predisposition, but where the relative contribution of this versus environmental factors has not yet been worked out. Also, in these situations, one is frequently dealing not just with one clearly defective gene but with an unfavourable constellation of several different genes. Human genetics in general cannot yet provide useful advice in these more complex situations.

Let us revert now to those clear-cut situations in which a known, bad gene is recessive, i.e. where GB individuals are healthy but BB individuals are sick. The latter will be diagnosed by the normal processes of clinical medicine, and accuracy of genetic diagnosis will depend on the state of medical knowledge concerning the particular bad trait or gene. We shall consider in some detail the role of routine health screening, which could add to the number of BB persons picked up. The carrier, phenotypically G but genotypically GB, present a bigger problem. How does a person know that he is a carrier of a particular bad trait? Frequently, the recessive gene is not completely silent. It causes no major upset but disturbs bodily chemistry in a minor way. The biochemical abnormality can then be picked up by sensitive and specialized laboratory tests. As there are many different genetic diseases, and as the tests are specific to particular traits and quite expensive, it is clearly not feasible at the present time to screen whole populations for all known carrier state abnormalities, though this might become possible at some time in the future. At present, carriers are identified in a rather *ad hoc* manner by studies of relatives of people with the frank disease, or, rarely, by limited population surveys sponsored by a research group with a particular interest in that genetic trait. What they choose to do about having children is then a matter for them to decide, after appropriate genetic counselling.

## Genetic counselling

I have said that human genetics is making rapid progress, but it would be equally fair to say that it is a subject not yet known in great detail to most practicing doctors. Many of the hereditary diseases are rare, and, as we have already admitted, the exact contribution of genetics to some diseases is still controversial and not understood in detail. The job of giving genetic advice to couples who have occasion to be worried (for example if they have had an abnormal child or if there is a family history of some illness) is one for a specialist in human genetics. The name we give to his duties in advising people is genetic counselling. This is becoming a recognized and important medical field, and is usually regarded as a sub-specialty of paediatrics (child health). In many communities, the existence of a competent genetic counsellor is not sufficiently well-known because of the newness of the specialty, and couples receive less informed advice as a result.

The counsellor makes it his job to keep up with all available literature and statistics about genetic disorders, and to know about any new special test for the detection of carriers. Where possible, he will brief couples on risk factors, and about the gravity or otherwise of the genetic anomaly. In some cases, his role becomes a more active one, because of the possibility of genetic testing of unborn children.

## Application of human genetics to embryos

Let us take the case of a known recessive genetic trait present in both parents. They have given birth to a defective child that has died or been placed into an institution, and they wish to have another child. The chances are one in four for another affected child, two in four for a healthy child but itself a carrier, and one in four for a healthy child not of carrier status. At present, there is no way of selecting sperms or eggs for possession of the good or the bad gene. If the couple wish a pregnancy, they must take their chances. However, in some cases, the genetic status of the unborn child can be determined in the womb. This is still only possible for a minority of genetic disorders, some seventy in all, but the relevant technology is advancing and spreading. The diagnostic test is not entirely without risk. It involves passing a thin, hollow needle through the mother's abdomen under local anaesthetic. This penetrates successively the abdominal wall and the wall of the womb (uterus) and reaches the fluid layer (amniotic fluid) in which the developing embryo leads its cosy cushioned existence. A small amount of the amniotic fluid is withdrawn, and the relevant genetic, microscopic or biochemical test is performed. Complications are infrequent, but include haemorrhage or miscarriage.

The results of the test are obtained quite quickly, and, depending on the social, religious and aesthetic convictions of the parents, a decision is made whether to terminate pregnancy. This at present is more frequently done for affected children but might in the future be considered also for carriers. One problem with this approach is that the fluid-tapping technique, known as amniocentesis, is only technically feasible at 14 to 16 weeks gestation, a period much further along than is ideal for medical termination of pregnancy.

It is clear that this whole area of human genetics, counselling and active termination of pregnancy for eugenic reasons raises some deep issues for society. I have gone into the subject in some detail, because it exemplifies the kind of social problem that medical science can bring forward. There are many similar ones, and the need for dialogue between the medical profession and society on these issues is becoming acute. Apart from ethical and moral considerations, there are enormous legal implications in many of these new developments.

One variant on the above theme is by now reasonably well known. Certain viruses can cross from the pregnant woman to the unborn child via the bloodstream and the placenta. The best studied example is the rubella (german measles) virus. When the virus gets access to the delicate tissues of the embryo, and particularly during the vital period of eight to twelve weeks gestation as the various organs are forming, it can cause severe damage resulting in serious birth defects such as blindness, deafness, or abnormality of the heart. Antibody tests on the mother can now confirm the german measles diagnosis. It is not yet possible to tell whether the embryo has 'caught' the disease, but medical termination of pregnancy on the basis of an unacceptably high risk of an abnormal baby is now widely accepted. In fact, some communities have passed relevant legislation.

The situation is more complex with some other viruses, such as measles or certain influenza strains, where the possibility has been raised of potential for foetal damage, but where the risk factors are obviously much smaller. In general, termination is not advised in the present state of medical knowledge.

The whole question of birth defects is receiving greatly increased attention since the tragic thalidomide story. In 1961 my Australian colleague Dr. William McBride first became suspicious about thalidomide when he noted, in a letter to 'The Lancet', that two doctors' wives had given birth to children with serious defects in the growth of their upper limbs. The only fact in common between them was that they had both taken the new sleeping pill, not yet widely available in Australia. McBride's work was soon confirmed through an extensive survey by Lenz in Germany, and since then there has been a salutory degree of caution exercised with respect to taking drugs of any kind in early pregnancy. Apart from drugs and viruses, other causes of foetal damage include faulty chromosomes and antibodies made by the mother against cells of the child under some circumstances. However, the cause in many, perhaps the majority, of cases of birth defect remains unknown.

## Algeny

So far in this chapter, we have kept our feet planted firmly on the ground and have confined our attention to recent, real discoveries. We must now face some future prospects. Perhaps the most controversial of them is the possibility of chemical manipulation of man's genetic machinery – what Joshua Lederberg has termed algeny, or alchemy of the genes. Will it ever be possible to 'fix up' genetic defects by chemical manipulations? Will one have the capacity to introduce into a human embryo some desirable characteristic, such as high intelligence? The background to this question comes from the world of genetics of very simple life forms, such as bacteria. These are single-celled organisms that normally divide by simple splitting into two, although we now know that a process akin to sexual reproduction (or sharing of genetic information between two bacteria resulting in changed progeny) does occur occasionally. Scientists are now good at creating and keeping alive all kinds of bizarre, defective mutants of bacteria, that could never survive in the wild. These act as useful models for study of genetic processes. A number of techniques are available by which such genetic defects can be cured. For example, certain viruses have the capacity to grow inside bacteria. One can make a virus grow in a 'good' bacterium and then ask it to carry a piece of 'good' DNA to the 'bad' mutant. The virus inserts this into the defective mutant and, in a certain percentage of cases, the genetic defect is fixed up and 'healthy' bacterial progeny result. This process is termed transduction. Alternatively, one can soak bacteria in preparations of purified DNA and obtain a percentage of bacteria carrying the genetic information absorbed from the surroundings. This process is called bacterial transformation.

Can transduction and transformation be applied to that very special single-celled organism, the human sperm? The answer is: not yet, and perhaps not for many decades or centuries. The reasons relate largely to the fact that bacteria are rapidly growing organisms which divide once every twenty minutes or so, whereas spermatozoa do not divide at all. The techniques of bacterial genetics depend on this growth, both for the detection of mutants in the first place, and for the production and detection of 'cured' bacteria after the transduction or transformation process. I do not wish to become too technical here, but for non-reproducing organisms a whole new conceptual and technologic framework would have to be built. Neither transduction nor transformation are efficient processes; under the best circumstances, some two per cent of bacteria exposed would be correctly altered. The detection of this sub-population in the absence of the amplifying mechanism of cell division in selective media would require a microchemical technology of quite formidable dimensions.

Another aspect that must be borne in mind, is that mammalian cells are at least a thousand times more complex than bacterial cells. The whole question of the 'good' DNA getting to the right spot is orders of magnitude more complex. Nevertheless, in the field of immunology, there have been some claims that genetic transformation has been achieved in antibody-forming cells, although these claims have not been fully confirmed or accepted.

Considerable excitement has been occasioned by a report published in October, 1971, by Dr. Carl R. Merril and collaborators in the prestigious journal, 'Nature'. These workers grew in the test tube certain cells (called fibroblasts) from a patient with a particular enzyme defect. They then infected this tissue culture with a virus that had grown on bacterial cells possessing a healthy or normal form of the same enzyme. They have presented evidence that successful transduction did, in fact, take place. The infected culture began to manufacture 'good' enzyme, indicating that the enzyme defect had been 'cured'. The change was heritable through 40 days of culture, suggesting that the 'good' viral gene had been stably incorporated into the genetic material of the human cell. In the same issue, 'Nature' ran an editorial which stated that if the results could be independently confirmed, they would revolutionize genetic thinking. 'Nature' warned readers that they would find their minds flooding with scepticism and prejudice; in fact, the experiments appeared to have been very well designed and executed. Even if the revolutionary claims can be substantiated, there is still a gap between the test tube finding and a clinical application in man. Still, it must be admitted that the gap is an order of magnitude smaller than it would be without Merril's finding.

Let us not leap to the conclusion that algeny is at hand. We do not know whether we shall be able to correct single gene defects as Merril hopes. Genetic traits such as intelligence, which are controlled by multiple genes and are much more vaguely understood, should not yet even enter into discussion of this topic. Nevertheless, the incredible strides of molecular biology have made 'never' or 'impossible' words that one hesitates to use.

## Cell fusion, cell culture and test-tube babies

Algeny is not the only form of major incursion into human breeding patterns that could be envisaged. There are several areas of modern cell biology that have at least the theoretical potential of human applicability in the short to medium term. Let us consider a few examples. In a number of animal species, it is now possible to induce division and maturation of female egg cells by means other than fertilization with a sperm. In other words, offspring result that have a mother but no father. These so-called 'parthogenetic' progeny are not all identical to the mother, as there is heterogeneity amongst the different eggs of the one female in terms of the genes they contain. However, there is one variant on this theme, so far practicable only for amphibia, where a series of identical twin-like replicas of an individual can be made. In this technique, the nucleus containing the DNA of the egg cell is removed surgically or destroyed by irradiation. Then, by microsurgery, a nucleus from some other cell, for example an intestine-lining cell, is injected into the enucleated egg. In about two per cent of cases, the 'operation' is successful and the egg goes on to divide and produce a tadpole and eventually a frog or toad. If a series of ten transplanted nuclei all come from the same animal, then ten genetically identical offspring would result, all being genetically identical to the donor of the nuclei.

Once again, the step from amphibian model to human application is a considerable one. However, on this occasion, far fewer bridges would have to be crossed than in the case of algeny. If a large enough team of scientists, given extensive powers over human guinea-pigs set themselves the task of producing replicas of Brigitte Bardot or President Kennedy, they could probably achieve their goal within ten years. Some of the steps would involve ghoulish concepts. The eggs would have to be harvested from the ovaries of women about to ovulate (i.e. at about the middle of the menstrual cycle) by operation. The surgically-fertilized eggs could be grown for a short time in the test tube, but would soon have to be transplanted into the womb of a woman pre-treated with hormones to put her into a pseudo-pregnant state. A mad dictator, willing to put up with the virtually inevitable crop of failures, leading to miscarriages and deformed babies, would have to be necessary before this scenario took place. However, being more realistic, it seems likely that such procedures will be possible in the mouse within a few years.

Other wonders, approaching science-fiction dimensions, can also be mentioned briefly. In the mouse, it is now possible to take two very young embryos from two different pregnant mice, and to place them into tissue culture in such a way that the two little embryos merge and fuse into one. This is done at a stage *before* organs, limbs and so forth have developed. Thus the end-result of the procedure is not like Siamese twins, it is something more foreign and frightening. The fused mass of embyonic tissue is implanted into the womb of a pseudo-pregnant foster-mother. Again with a certain number of failures, the experiment ends with the natural birth of a perfectly-formed little mouse with *two* fathers and *two* mothers. Half its cells are from one set of parents; half from a second, forming what is termed a mosaic. The two sets of cells seem to live in perfect harmony with each other. If the two sets of parent mice are of different colours, the mosaic mouse product turns out a striped mixture. This is a readily visible sign of mosaicism, and more technical tests have established that the same holds true for internal organs. One cannot see any advantage in having people generated in this way; the example is cited chiefly to illustrate what can already be done in cell biology applied to mammalian reproduction.

Another exciting research area is in the field of fusion of actual mammalian cells. If certain tricks are used to glue two cells together, they will merge and join in much the way that two oil globules will do so. The resultant hybrid cell will have a double lot of genetic information, and is a useful tool in working out nuclear-cytoplasmic relationships and other aspects of the inner workings of cells. There are some who hope that it might one day be possible to fuse cancer cells in the body with some injected cell that 'teaches the cancer cell to be good again', but once more we are in the realm of the far-fetched here.

We have mentioned growing embryos in test tubes for short periods. Will it be possible to produce test-tube babies? So far, efforts to keep embryos nourished in test tubes have succeeded best for very young embryos, that require to be fed only by the process of diffusion. Later on, nutrition of the foetus depends on availability of foodstuffs from the mother transported via a complex and important structure called the afterbirth or placenta. Some experimentation is going on concerning 'feeding' of animal foetuses by artificial fluids and oxygenating them by pumps of various sorts. As the problems of keeping even one kidney alive for more than a couple of days has not yet been solved, it will be a long time before the problems of correctly feeding a growing embryo will yield to technology. This again is one of those research areas of the more applied kind where rate of progress depends largely and directly on amount of effort expended, and most scientists would agree that this is an area not deserving of high priority.

Determination of sex of the unborn child is a topic that has long fascinated mankind. Amniocentesis can now achieve this knowledge and theoretically abortion could be performed if the sex of the embryo were not the one wanted. Will one ever be able to induce a planned male or female pregnancy? Determination of the sex of a child depends on whether the sperm brings an *x* or a *y* chromosome to the egg, which always has an *x* chromosome. In the latter case, the infant will be *xy*, and male; in the former, *xx* and female. Theoretically the *y*-carrying sperms, which have a little less DNA in them than the *x* carrying ones, ought to be able to be separated by some biophysical trick. This is not yet possible, but one day it could well be. In that case, a pool of sperms from the husband could be fractionated into 'male' and 'female' types, and the wife could be artificially inseminated with the one or the other. In a society becoming increasingly aware of the need for population control, there might be a real desire on the part of many couples to have just one boy and one girl as their total family. In contrast to many of the examples considered above, there is nothing gruesome involved in any of the sequential steps of the contemplated procedure. It would not surprise me to see the facility for this type of 'birth control' become available within ten to fifteen years.

## Control of cellular differentiation

It is well known that many lower vertebrate species can regenerate substantial portions of their body if these are cut off. In man, however, the potential for regeneration is much more limited. Those tissues which normally 'turn over', i.e. die and are reborn, exhibit great powers of recuperation. Blood loss can be made good; burnt skin heals over if the damage is not too deep; cut hair grows; and broken bones mend. However, regeneration in the sense of regrowth of an amputated digit or limb does not occur, and the most important cells of all, the nerve cells of the brain, cannot regrow if killed by injury or disease. In fact, division of nerve cells in the brain stops at two years of age in the human. The best that can happen is that some other portion of the brain takes over the function of a part that is lost.

The process governing growth of cells and assumption of specialized functions by cells is called differentiation. Overall, although we have accurate descriptive knowledge of many aspects of differentiation, the underlying biochemical mechanisms are still largely obscure. We do know, however, that growth of some types of cells is controlled by chemical molecules made by other cells. Some of these growth-stimulating factors have been isolated and partially purified. For example, there are molecules that stimulate certain still-growing nerve cells in very young animals; others that cause growth of white blood cells. Drs. D. Metcalf and E. R. Stanley at my Institute are making rapid progress in the purification of factors in the last-named group, and are learning a great deal about their mode of action.

Many authorities believe that a study of differentiation will represent one of the next big glamour fields in biomedical research. It is relevant to many problems in practical medicine: birth control; birth defects; cancer; repair of injury; retardation of ageing, and others. If a massive effort in research on differentiation, say in the 1980's, is crowned with the same success as that which is apparent and likely for immunology over the period 1960 – 1980, the face of medical practice may be altered in ways that we dare not dream of yet.

## Neurobiology, psychiatry and mind control

There is a curious parallel between differentiation and neurobiology, the study of the nervous system including the brain. In both cases, we have a wealth of descriptive phenomenology, a wonderfully detailed knowledge of certain fragments, but an absence of the kind of total insight that would add up to an acceptable general theory. In this respect the two fields are behind, for example, molecular biology or immunology. Fortunately, in both cases, the restricted internal methodology proper to the field itself is now being augmented by a veritable onslaught of techniques and concepts derived from other disciplines in biology. In particular, newer methods of biochemistry and cell biology are being brought to bear on the key issues.

As regards brain research, these fundamental efforts have not yet begun to pay off in a clinical sense. As we have seen in Chapter 3, there has been a revolution in clinical psychiatry, but this has resulted from an empirical approach rather than from pure science. Indeed, there has been quite a paradoxical situation here, as the empiric discovery of certain drugs that ameliorate psychotic states was a big stimulus to research on chemical aspects of nerve impulse transmission in the central nervous system. In turn, of course, better information on nerve transmitter substances has helped the search for better drugs, and thus the reaction becomes circular. The end result as seen at the present time is that, though we do not understand the fundamental causes of mental illnesses, we have a battery of drugs that can give dramatic symptomatic relief in many cases, and that are an invaluable help to rehabilitation and occasionally even to cure of grave mental illnesses.

Inevitably, this capacity to control abnormal states such as manic excitement, severe depression or withdrawal from reality as occurs in schizophrenia, raises the issue of whether it would be possible to use similar techniques to control the minds of normal people. In my opinion, the possibility is real. We already have a variety of drugs that can affect mood, lessen or increase inhibitions, distort reality, reduce energy and drive, and so forth. It is a tragic thing to see these powerful pharmacological agents, most of which were developed by medical science for specific useful purposes, abused by the 'hippie' subculture and by other rebels or misfits. The human dilemma is a great one; the temptation to opt out a real one for many; but the fact remains that the man-made mess can only be cleaned up, or at least prevented from deteriorating further, by disciplined human effort. No drug has yet been discovered that can consistently and over a period improve the performance of a healthy, normal human in any task. Arguing from a teleological standpoint, this is for the very good reason that, if such a drug did exist, nature would have discovered it first and used it to improve the species. The argument may be specious, but the observation that drugs are harmful if given to normal people is still a valid generalization. In other words, my view is that to contemplate mass use of drugs for mind control as part of some wide social purpose is incredibly dangerous and mischievous thinking. One can but hope that this aspect of Aldous Huxley's thinking remains in the realm of fiction for ever.

It may be more profitable to consider other types of mind control. Certainly the kind of social indoctrination that appears to be part of the Chinese communist educational system is a powerful force in shaping society. I have not had occasion to read much of the technical literature on 'brainwashing' experiments, but it appears that a great deal can be achieved without the use either of drugs or of physical force. There is a large grey area between biological science, behavioural science and educational psychology here that needs to be much better defined. This hardly falls within the scope of the present book, but it does illustrate the importance of human biology in very practical terms.

## Genetics, intelligence and race

In many ways we have in the last two chapters, been tending to look at man as if he were a machine. Of course to an extent man is a piece of biological machinery, but in a way that so far totally eludes medical science, he is also much more. At present, the techniques of medical biology are good at understanding the *similarities* between man and animals, but they are not yet very good at understanding the *differences*. The behavioural sciences and the humanities must help us here. A great controversy has arisen in recent years over inherent, overall genetically predetermined differences in intelligence and human capability amongst the different races. This has reached its most disturbing form in the United States, where the question is whether the black man is genetically inferior to the white. It is easy to get emotional about this problem. I have had occasion to discuss it with many scientists expert in genetics and sociology. There is no doubt that the overwhelming weight of informed opinion is against the view of Dr. Shockley, who believes the black man's inferiority has been proven. The big point is: what do IQ tests measure? Apart from inherent capacity of brain cells, there are extremely relevant variables in education, experience, motivation, habit and discipline that modify human performance. It is a well-known rule in science that any experiment is only as good as the techniques used in it. If a substance is unmeasurable by present technology, there is no point in yet pursuing rigorous scientific work depending on accurate quantitation of that substance. Therefore, there is no point arguing about the relevant *potential* of one group of humans versus another, as the techniques for measuring this overall potential are so primitive. It is much more worthwhile to expend ones energies on devising social patterns which encourage greater expression of human potential by *all* undereducated, under-privileged segments of society.

## Importance of education in human biology

This chapter has looked rather superficially at some aspects of the long-range capacity of molecular and cell biology for modification of human health, behaviour and evolution. I am conscious of having adopted a rather conservative line as regards the future. This is for two reasons. First, there are just too many publications that foreshadow extraordinary and revolutionary developments, without paying much heed to the need for responsibility. Secondly, I believe the speed of progress in this more futuristic area of medical biology will be slower than that in nuclear physics during the 1930's. The gap between the model systems and the real life situation in man is great indeed. Nevertheless, there will be progress, and there will be greatly increased power to interfere in natural processes. This power can be used for good or for evil; alternatively, as has been the case over the last twenty-seven years with respect to atomic and hydrogen bombs, mankind can elect not to use the power it possesses or will shortly possess.

In the case of physics, it turned out that a pleading for greater community awareness would have been irrelevant to the events that actually took place. Progress was just too rapid for general education to have had a chance to play a role. In biology, progress has been and will continue to be great. I predict, however, that the pace will be somewhat less headlong than that in physics. If this turns out to be so, a pleading for wide community education in human biology and related biosciences may be effective in leading to the creation of a civilization that can master the advances as they come forward, rather than being mastered by them. This does not imply a desire to force a lot of technical detail on people. It is simply a wish to expose people to the broad general principles of man's make-up, and to the implications of these for the future, both immediate and remote. Such general community involvement would be the best insurance I can think of against the misuse of biological knowledge by some sub-segment of society. An informed, aware population giving a somewhat critical backing to its bioscientists will harness the forces they unleash to better ends.

*Further reading*

Burnet, F. M. *Genes, Dreams and Realities.* Medical and Technical Publishing Co. Ltd., Aylesbury (1971).

Huxley, J. *What Dare I Think?* Chatto and Windus, London (1931).

Leach, G. *The Biocrats.* Jonathan Cape, London (1970).

Medawar, P. B. *The Uniqueness of the Individual.* Methuen and Co. Ltd., London (1957).

# 11

# Computers and automation in medicine

'*That it will ever come into general use notwithstanding its value, is extremely doubtful; because its beneficial application requires much time and gives a good bit of trouble to the patient and practitioner.*' London Times, 1834, commenting on Laennec's introduction of the stethoscope.

Computers have revolutionized many aspects of science, industry and the professions. The computer's incredible speed and accuracy in making sequential, contingent 'yes – no' decisions, combined with its capacity to deal logically with virtually unlimited amounts of information, have allowed man to tackle problems in a manner that would otherwise have been inconceivable. The computer's dominant role in space exploration, national defence systems, government and banking has been the subject of public amusement, bewilderment and admiration in countless films and novels. Information and computing science is one of the newest, largest and still most rapidly growing branches of modern learning. All of this is common knowledge but what is less often talked about is the fact that the two greatest professions, medicine and the law, have been the last to come to real grips with the computer age. Biomedical computation does exist as a field, but relative to its long-range importance, it is at a very primitive stage of development.

Medical decision-making, that is reaching a diagnosis, planning treatment and making judgements about likely outcome of disease in an individual patient, is at the centre of medical practice. The improvement of medical decision-making is the long-range goal of medical research. It might be supposed that the basis of medical decision-making is logic, and that the processes involved are clear-cut and well understood. Surprisingly enough, we do not really know much about the detailed mental processes by which a doctor reaches a diagnosis. There certainly are elements of logical deduction involved, but 'intuition' and 'seat of the pants feeling' may sometimes play a role. As medicine becomes more scientific, so there is a need for greater precision in diagnosis, and indeed for more rigorous definition of disease states.

The long-range goal of harnessing the computer as an aid to medical decision-making would be to improve decisions through greater knowledge of disease. If the knowledge and experience of many doctors could be pooled, and the certitude of the computer's memory substituted for the frailties of human memory, many aspects of medical care would become more exact. Predictions as to success or otherwise of treatment would be based on extensive statistics; the likely results of treatment options would be available on a probability basis; drug evaluation could be based on much more complex, multifactorial analysis; research into correlations between different factors in disease causation would be facilitated. It is no exaggeration to say that the fabric of clinical research would be revolutionized. Therefore, why is this not happening? The reasons for this are manifold, but most of them can be included in four words: conservatism, communication, cost, complexity.

## Difficulties in biomedical computation

The medical profession is, by its very nature, conservative. It is faced with responsibilities over life and death that would be almost unbearable for an individual if not backed by an established, venerated set of customs and beliefs. In fact, medicine can only progress when individuals use tradition as their springboard for more imaginative leaps into the unknown. Traditionalism can, unfortunately, easily merge into inertia. It can also be accompanied by a certain fear and mistrust of the unknown. I think it is fair to say that many medical men fear automation and computers, either sensing rivals to their own self-assumed omnipotence and omniscience, or harbouring doubts about depersonalization of medical practice. The proponent of computers in medicine thus begins with a handicap – rather than facing a strictly neutral audience, he has to deal with one that is a little uneasy and resentful.

Communication between information scientist and doctor is also difficult. There is a great deal of mutual ignorance about each other's activities. In my experience, the information scientist has an oversimplified view of medicine, whereas the doctor's knowledge of computer science, even in the sketchiest outline, is virtually non-existent. Clearly a medical information system could only be generated through a thorough-going collaboration between the two camps, and in practical terms, this is not easy to achieve.

The cost factor in setting up a viable research project in bio-medical computation is considerable. Even if hospital-wide systems might eventually save large sums of money and greatly increase efficiency, they must be preceded by years of expensive and initially non-productive development work, which would add further to the spiralling costs of hospitals. In particular, unless computer 'hardware' is available from some other source, such as an affiliated university, this item will loom frighteningly large on the budget. It could be argued that the costs could be amalgamated into the construction costs of a new hospital, which are usually reckoned in the many millions of dollars, but the problem is that blueprints for a really effective medical information system do not exist anywhere in the world. There have been many fragmentary advances, and a great deal of talk, but a 'medical decision-making machine' in the full sense does not exist.

This brings us to to the fourth point, that of the complexity of the problem. There are literally thousands of different diseases, and some hundreds of reasonably common ones. There are many hundreds of different specialized laboratory diagnostic tests. There are several thousands of specific questions which one might wish to ask to elicit a full and exact medical history. The number of permutations and combinations of treatment options is virtually infinite. In some respects it can be claimed that no two patients are exactly alike. The job of so structuring and formalizing medical information as to render it capable of being handled by computer is therefore very great indeed.

In my Institute, we have nevertheless set ourselves the task of creating a medical information system based on computers. The task has not been easy, and is by no means finished. However, results to date have been so encouraging that it may be worthwhile summarizing the highlights in this chapter. The work to which I will refer has been largely performed by Drs. V. X. Gledhill and J. D. Mathews, with some preliminary work by Dr. T. A. McPherson, and under the overall supervision of Dr. I. R. Mackay.

## The three major divisions of medical information

Any computational approach to disease must have reliable data on which to feed, and we decided quite early in the piece that the formal record of a patient's illness must be the data base. The medical record is the document which charts the patient's progress from first encounter with the doctor through till eventual cure or death. It should have all the information necessary for efficient patient management and for subsequent research into that particular condition. It is a document of great legal, medical and educational importance. In a doctor's consulting rooms, the records may be rather rudimentary, the doctor relying on his memory to supply needed detail, but in a hospital, the records must be comprehensive, as they may be the only means of maintaining continuity of patient management when residents change shift, or when illnesses run on for long periods.

Each medical record will have in it three types of primary information, together with such conclusions as might be derived from this. First, there is the medical *history*: a listing of the patient's complaints, both major and minor, and of his responses to interrogation. Secondly comes the physical examination, where the doctor examines the patient for abnormalities that he can see, or hear, or feel, using his hands, eyes and a few simple instruments such as the stethoscope, ophthalmoscope, knee-jerk hammer, etc. Thirdly, as a result of cogitating on the data generated by these two means, the doctor may order some diagnostic tests, the results of which are also inserted into the medical record. Physically, the medical record consists of a loose-leaf binder, more frequently handwritten rather than typed, of greatly variable length (minimum about 4 pages up to a maximum of many hundreds of pages for a complex case with multiple hospital admissions) averaging perhaps 20 pages, though this will depend on the type of patient. We must consider each of the three types of record in some detail.

## The medical history

The medical history is traditionally regarded as the most important part of the information related to a patient's disease. All medical students are taught that they must spend a great deal of time listening to the patient describing the symptoms which occasioned him to consult a doctor. First, the patient must be allowed to tell it all in his own words, and then the picture must be rounded out by gently interrogating the patient about his disease, carefully avoiding posing too many leading questions. It has frequently been claimed that, on the basis of history alone, one can tell whether the patient has a duodenal ulcer, or gall-stones, or pancreatitis. The crushing or burning pain in the chest typical of coronary artery disease *is* quite different in character from the sharp, stabbing pain with local tenderness characteristic of pleurisy. In other words, there is probably much substance to the idea that a good history is the cornerstone of good clinical medicine.

There are a number of factors, however, which modify this picture. First and foremost is the question of time. In general practice there is rarely time to take a full medical history. It is usually stated that a first interview with a patient (including the physical examination) should take about one hour, and even in consultant practice this is not easily achieved. In hospital, residents may or may not have the time to take a good history. In either case, the job is usually delegated to the most junior member of the hospital team, who may be rather prone to 'lead' the patient in a direction that the text-books have set out, and the history can come out rather like a stereotyped version of the history that *should* accompany the disease which the resident thinks the patient might have. Often the resident does do a good job in taking the history, but in order for this information to be of real use to the senior specialist when he comes to see the case, it must be legible and not too diffuse or lengthy. Few specialists have the time to wade through reams of accurate description of symptoms, particularly as they will frequently wish to retake at least portions of the history in their own way.

Perhaps the biggest problem of all in the usual hand-written free format history is the difficulty of using it in any efficient way for the furtherance of medical knowledge. Suppose that an investigator wished to establish in what proportion of cases the pain of an ulcer worked its way from the abdomen through to the back. He would have to go to the medical library, take down from the shelves the files of all patients with duodenal ulcer, and thumb through the history until he found (or did not find!) the handwritten description of the nature of the pain. This very simple example of a medical record search would take a good number of hours. More realistic research projects become major enterprises with the present record system, and clinicians who have tried their hand at this type of retrospective clinical analysis become more and more disenchanted with present record systems. Illegibility and incompleteness are the most frequent complaints.

Gledhill and Mathews have devised a computer approach to the medical history which avoids all these problems, though it may offend the traditionalist and may require supplementation for immediate management of the patient. The project is termed SASH, an acronym for self-administered symptom history.

### SASH – A two-stage process for obtaining medical history information in machine-processable form

The principle of SASH is that the patient gives his medical history essentially as a series of 'yes – no' answers to a set of medical questions. It does not have the same disadvantage of 'leading the witness', as *all* patients, regardless of their disease, get the same primary list of questions, 284 in number, to which they must respond. The patient ticks off 'yes' or 'no', and the results are fed to the computer, which generates a patient-individualized secondary questionnaire. This asks more detailed, searching questions about those symptoms which the patient ticked off as positive. For example, if the patient checks off 'yes' to the question: 'In the past year, have you had a bad headache?', the computer will print out a list of questions relating to the frequency, duration, character, exact location, severity, etc. of that headache. Naturally, the length of the secondary questionnaire will depend on how many items of the primary questionnaire are checked off as positive. The available list of questions from which the secondary questionnaire was generated numbered over 4000.

Once the patient has completed the secondary questionnaire, the responses are again fed into the computer. It then converts this coded list of numbers into sentences of medical English, and prints out a history in narrative form very similar in its overall style to the history taken and recorded by physicians themselves. Of course, all the codified information in the history is stored in the computer in the much simpler and shorter form of a string of numbers. The translated form of the history is not only very readable, but much more complete than the history usually taken by residents. It often draws attention to a problem area, for example in the psychological or sexual field, which the patient might not spontaneously reveal to the doctor. Of course, the system is not perfect. It can be foiled by stupidity or carelessness of the patient. It may be tricked by malingerers or hypochondriacs, though it is not at present self-evident that the computer is more easily fooled by these than the doctor. In fact, it may be that a 'symptom profile' very characteristic of these groups, or of psychoneurotic patients, will emerge. Finally, SASH may miss nuances that may require further exploration when the patient is interviewed.

One big advantage of SASH is that it can be generated in the total absence of the doctor. The physician's time is one of the most expensive items in health care delivery and, in many places, still one of the scarcest. Under ideal circumstances a non-urgent case would not actually see the doctor until both stages of SASH had been completed. The doctor could then see the patient with the full history already laid out.

The permanence and ready accessibility of this codified history data represent even more important advantages. A record search for frequency or coincidental presence of any number of symptoms becomes quite a trivial exercise, for, when such a system is fully set up, it would take only a matter of minutes.

It might be argued that SASH deprives the doctor and patient of the chance of forming a good relationship during the initial interview. In fact, the contrary appears to be the case. Precious time, that was previously taken up by asking a lot of questions and recording the answers in longhand, can now be spent in a more pleasant and social contact with the patient. Specific interrogation, instead of necessarily being directed at umbrella-like coverage, can be deep and searching about aspects revealed by SASH. Most patients actually love doing SASH and find themselves fascinated by the process. Most physicians have been surprised at the completeness and acceptable nature of the SASH write-back.

Many physicians argue that a history based on a questionnaire cannot possibly convey the shades of meaning and description that a personal interview can reveal. This may be true, but we must ask whether there is not an exaggerated respect for the subtlties of the medical history, that has grown out of tradition rather than hard scientific fact. How often is the *definitive* diagnosis of duodenal ulcer made on the basis of the nature of the abdominal pain? Is it not generally accepted that the final court of appeal is more likely to be the barium meal X-ray examination? Moreover, the traditional history is of little value for research, as anyone who has had the task of searching through some hundreds of typical hospital histories will readily agree. Finally, there is no theoretical limit to the completeness obtainable by automated techniques. A group especially interested in headache or cardiac pain could easily devise a further and still more detailed questionnaire to be completed by relevant patients.

SASH generates a symptom profile for each given patient. As we shall see, this forms part of the data base from which the computer will eventually be asked to make a medical diagnosis. Physical examination and special tests obviously also contribute to this.

## Physical examination check list (PECL)

The physical examination conducted by the doctor in order to detect lumps, rashes, tenderness, heart murmurs and the like, is usually more 'structured' than the history-taking. Most hospitals have set requirements in this regard, with lists of specific things that must be looked for and recorded. Accordingly, the physical examination lends itself rather readily to a computer approach. Gledhill and Mathews had little difficulty in generating a physical examination check list (PECL), where residents could record, in considerable detail, their list of abnormal findings. Again, it is not possible to examine in detail every system of the body, and the check-list provided for recording in two stages. Further, a facility whereby the computer prints out the results in acceptable medical English, is again included. One virtue of the system is that it ensures that when a particular examination (e.g. a detailed examination of the nervous system) has *not* been performed, the resident is required to check a square that states so. In other words, the record is more complete than the usual hand-written one. Moreover, the residents find the printed sheets where abnormal findings must be recorded a useful aide-memoire for their physical examination, and, for the most part, appreciate not having to write out a long, detailed description. Once the residents have become accustomed to the forms, PECL, though very comprehensive, actually saves time.

### Computer handling of special tests

The special laboratory tests which are so frequently necessary to confirm a medical diagnosis are normally ordered on the basis of a working hypothesis or provisional diagnosis that the doctor reaches as a result of history and physical examination. The computer can learn to recognize what constellation of symptoms and signs require particular diagnostic tests, and can produce a list of desirable tests. This can be checked by the resident for what he may believe to be errors of omission or commission. We believe that as the number of cases processed by computer increases, its judgement about provisional diagnosis on the basis of SASH and PECL will improve, and that it will be a useful aid to the resident in ordering tests. It may even be that this could save money. At present, residents tend to over-order tests, as they do not want to be caught out when the senior physician comes on his ward round and asks whether this or that test has been performed. If the ordering of a test must be justified on objective criteria, actually fewer tests might be performed. One could envisage that a resident might be required to justify in a special way tests not ordered by the computer.

The results of many tests could be handled by the computer without any problem. This applies to numeric results (level of haemoglobin in the blood, number of white cells, amount of sugar, etc), but some diagnostic tests result in data of a different sort. For example, an X-ray may reveal shadows in the lung that could represent tuberculosis, cancer or congestion due to heart failure. The radiologist may find features that are more suggestive of one of the three, but will often not be in a position to press his view dogmatically. In such cases, the diagnosis finally arrived at will depend on a balanced judgement involving other tests and the total clinical picture. From the viewpoint of biomedical computation, the X-ray picture could be entered into the record in several different ways. For example, the radiologist could be asked for his opinion with subjective weighting factors, e.g. 60% probability of tuberculosis, 30% of cancer, 10% of lung congestion. Alternatively, he could be required to check off the features of the X-ray according to some agreed check-list akin to PECL. In our computer project, this bridge remains to be crossed, but our general orientation is towards objectivity wherever possible.

## Diagnosis Profiles

A central feature of our system is that there should be continuing interaction between physician and computer. The computer can only learn the correlation between certain symptoms, physical abnormalities and results of laboratory tests, on the one hand, and specific diagnoses, on the other, if it is taught these correlations by doctors. In other words, for the first several thousand cases fed into the computer, the clinical diagnosis, arrived at by the physicians looking after the case, must be supplied so that the computer can construct a profile of symptoms, signs, and test results that constitute the statistical norms of each particular disease. The mathematics of this process are relatively simple. In due course, each symptom, sign and test result will be given a 'weighting factor' by the computer with respect to every disease of which the computer has experience. The computer can very rapidly scan the profile of a particular patient and compare it with the profiles of each disease. When it finds the best match, this gives the most likely diagnosis. It could also print out a list of progressively less likely diagnoses. Eventually, when the 'case memory' of the computer has built up to a sufficient degree, this diagnostic facility might be a useful decision-making aid to the physician. Obviously, the larger the bank of cases, the better will be the performance of the computer. If a learning system is properly programmed, the diagnostic facility would get better and better with the progress of time. One could envisage a number of hospitals pooling information for the extension and updating of diagnosis profiles. The case memory of a given doctor is limited and fallible. The case memory of the computer is, in principle, virtually infinitely expandable, and certainly not susceptible to the sorts of errors that human memories exhibit!

This somewhat idealized outline is still quite futuristic. In fact, we do not know how long it will take to accumulate the sort of case experience that could make the system effective. The initial cost will be substantial and unexpected pitfalls will undoubtedly be encountered on the way. Nevertheless, the progress already made in our laboratory has been heartening, and the final goal seems attainable.

## Biomedical computation and clinical research

Diagnosis by computer seems at first sight to be the most novel and glamorous application of computers to medicine. In fact, however, the establishment of a correct diagnosis is usually possible by conventional techniques. The rate-limiting factors in the progress of medicine are our lack of understanding of the causation of many diseases, and the ineffectiveness of many of the available treatments. Therefore, the question whether computers can help clinical research is even more important than their possible role in diagnosis. We believe strongly that they can help research of a certain type.

Much clinical research deals with correlations. The classic example is the association between smoking and lung cancer, which grew out of statistical, epidemiologic research. There are countless numbers of other examples. Is breast cancer more or less common in child-bearing women? It turns out that pregnancy has a certain protective effect especially if women have their first baby at a young age. Are gall-bladder patients really female, fair, fat and forty, as the text-books say? Is surgical or medical treatment better for ulcers? How often is pancreatitis due to alcoholism? How many patients who have a first epileptic fit at age forty in fact have a brain tumour? These are the sorts of issues that make up much of the day-to-day work of the clinical researcher, and hundreds if not thousands of papers are written each year, establishing or claiming some new, important correlation.

Multivariate analysis of this type is one of the things at which computers really excel. Mr. Jonathan Buckley in our laboratory has written a new computer language, called CLINTRAN, which allows access to our computer records. It is very simple to learn, and physicians would take only a day to become familiar with it. They can then do their own programming to ask any correlation they wish of the information stored in the computer's memory bank. In this way, work that would have taken months under the old medical record system can now be completed in half a day. The only problem is that the accumulation of case data for our computer system is a slow process, as there is no practical way of converting the old, existing records into the new, machine-processable format. However, if one can be patient enough to accumulate 3 to 5 years' worth of data, the research that one could do on the records generated over that time would be virtually limitless.

## Prognosis of disease

A sick person, and particularly one with family responsibilities, is naturally most anxious to be given information about the likely course of his disease. On presently-available treatment, what are the chances of death versus recovery, and what is the likely timing of each alternative? How much will capacity to work be affected? What are the relative risks inherent in different treatment options? This type of information together constitutes the prognosis of the case. At present, doctors tend to give prognoses in very vague terms. I am always amused by the description of medical prognoses in novels. So often one reads that: 'the doctor has given me 6 months to live' or 'I need two years to be cured'. In fact, in my experience, physicians are most reluctant to commit themselves to numbers of any sort, when giving a patient or a relative a case prognosis. They may indicate in a general way the likely outcome and the broad pace of disease progression, but the central question: 'Doctor, how long have I got?' is usually left unanswered. There are many reasons for this, some of them humanitarian and psychological, but one reason is ignorance. We simply do not have precise enough information on sufficiently large numbers of cases of many diseases to give the kind of statistical answer that should, theoretically, be possible. Here is another area where a computer-accessible data base would be invaluable.

The system developed at the Walter and Eliza Hall Institute, and more recently set up on a larger scale at the Royal Prince Alfred Hospital in Sydney by Dr. Gledhill, has been described in some detail. This is not meant in any sense to imply that it is unique. Many other efforts in the same general direction are in progress and some, particularly in the United States, United Kingdom and Sweden, are of much larger dimensions. Some of these are described in detail in the further reading listed on page 173.

## Greater objectivity and logic in medical care

One of the most striking fringe benefits which we have already observed at our Institute from the existence of a computer system is the tendency for greater objectivity, precision and logic in every aspect of medical care. When one knows that every statement, opinion, test request or treatment suggestion must be defended and justified, as it will form part of the computer's learning process, there is great pressure to conform to the highest scientific standards. One product of this process has been the development of the medical synopsis. This is a working document, compiled progressively by the medical staff. It is 'problem-oriented'; for each diagnosis (or as yet undiagnosed problem) there is a brief listing of relevant symptoms, physical signs, test results and present or recommended treatment. There is room also for a brief 'discharge opinion' that summarizes the head physician's overview of the case. While the patient is in hospital, the handwritten form of this synopsis presents a very handy summary of the current clinical status of the case, of use to consultants called in to see the patient, or to resident staff involved in the patient's care at nights or on weekends. At discharge, the synopsis is typed into the computer terminal, forming a permanent part of the case record. It can also be rearranged by the computer in a form suitable as a discharge summary, that can be mailed to the referring doctor who will look after the patient on his return home. In fact, this synopsis approach to clinical records actually does not require computers at all. The point is that its implementation was facilitated by the fact that the staff involved had become used to detailed, point by point, analyses of clinical data.

## Cost-benefit analysis of computer-based medical record storage and retrieval system

At the present time, no one can say whether a system such as the one described would be worth the cost of setting it up. It could be argued that eventually much money would be saved through the greater efficiency of hospitals in general. Residents would have less paper-work, and would do their jobs more meticulously and logically. Medical record libraries would require less space and staff. Better information processing could lead to fewer mix-ups and less time-wasting in hospitals. Nevertheless, there is no doubt that the initial costs would be high. Specialized staff with commercially valuable know-how would have to be employed, and expensive computer 'hardware' would have to be installed. Teething problems would abound and a double record system would probably have to operate for some years. An unfortunate point is that the real value of the system is unlikely to emerge from small, inexpensive pilot projects like our own, and that therefore a sizeable expenditure, essentially of a risk-taking nature, may be required so that enough data can enter the computer to make its performance a fair test of the principles involved. There is much to be said for a small number of research centres attacking the job with courage, because the longer we wait and the more complex and technical medicine becomes, the more formidable would the task be to begin.

## Automation of diagnostic tests

Striking progress has been made in other aspects of medical automation. Many biochemical and some haematological tests can be performed cheaply and efficiently by auto-analyzers of various types. While these are routine, other devices are still in the testing stage. For example, computers have been used for automatic analyses of heart and brain tests (electrocardiograms and electroencephalograms), or for determining the normality or otherwise of sets of chromosomes. In a research setting, many complex bits of apparatus are linked directly to computers. Properly used, this automation has greatly improved the output of both routine diagnostic and research laboratories. Unfortunately, once a test becomes cheap, there is a real danger of over-use, and the cost benefit of having each test done more cheaply is negated by many more tests being performed.

This leads us on naturally to the very controversial area known as multiphasic health screening. This concept requires that large masses of healthy people, or even whole populations, have regular, highly scientific health check-ups, involving not only clinical examinations but a battery of blood and other tests. The value of such an approach to medicine will be discussed in the next chapter. Let us document here that the issue comes up mainly because automation has made it possible. In Chapter 12, we shall also look more closely at the depersonalizing or dehumanizing aspect of computers and automation in medicine.

Reverting finally once more to research, I wish to conclude this chapter on a positive note. Computers in the clinic remain controversial. It may even turn out that our present hopes are over-optimistic; that we are promoting an idea the time of which has not yet come. However, the better processing of information by computers is already contributing notably to medical research. This is in the setting of automated literature search. There are a number of excellent computer systems, both government sponsored and private, which are fed the titles and other key-words of hundreds of thousands of research papers each year. They can help an investigator to obtain a listing of what work is going on in his area (i.e. according to keywords that he chooses), without demanding that he should search physically the tables of contents of hundreds or even thousands of technical journals. Ingenious variations on this theme have been developed. Computers can help an investigator to find any article which has had occasion to refer to his own work, and can thereby help him to judge what impact his work has had, or where his branch of science is heading in the opinion of his scientific peers. Information systems can send a scientist relevant technical articles or summaries thereof in the mail, obviating the need to subscribe to many journals that only occasionally print articles of interest to him. Again one forms the impression that this field of computer application is just beginning.

This chapter has probably shocked more people than any other, as the thought of a sick person being 'a case', just another statistic in a huge machine, does have its abhorrent aspect. Every person is a unique occurrence, and his health a uniquely important concern, at least to him. Intuitively, we regard our health in an intensely personal manner, and our relationship with our doctor as a special, very human one. Yet it is a central feature of science that it can deal only with reproducible events. Medical science can approach illness only after it has defined the commonality that links scores or hundreds or thousands of suffering human beings. The *common* features make it a case of diabetes, or schizophrenia, or cancer. The differences within a group of patients with one disease enlarge our understanding of that disease, and its possible range of symptoms and effects. The uniqueness of the actual patient who turns to his doctor for help is an aspect outside the science of medicine, but belonging to the ancient craft of medicine. It, too, is a precious and valuable aspect of medicine, and one which we must seek to preserve. We do not need to regard science and art as being joined in battle here. Both have their place.

*Further reading*

McLachlan, G. and Shegog, R. A. eds., *Computers in the Service of Medicine – essays on current research and applications*. Vols. I and II. Oxford University Press (1968).

Mason, E. E. and Bulgren, W. G. *Computer Applications in Medicine*. Charles C. Thomas, Springfield, III. (1964).

Rose, J. ed., *Proceedings of the Symposium on Computers in Medicine*. J. and A. Churchill Ltd. London (1969).

Stacey, R. W. and Waxman, B. eds., *Computers in Biomedical Research*. Academic Press, New York (1965).

# 12

# The impact of medical research on patterns of medical practice

'*Change must come; it can, on balance, be good; it is our business to try to guide it and ensure that it shall be not merely change but progress*'. Julian Huxley

The modern doctor faces almost daily a classic confrontation between two sides of his nature: that of the wise counsellor and healer; and that of the technically attuned biocrat. Let me illustrate what I mean by referring to two patients seen recently at the Walter and Eliza Hall Institute. The first was a lady of 75, in fair general health though distinctly frail, who complained of dizzy turns accompanied by faintness and at times by transient paralysis almost simulating a mild stroke. Questioning revealed that attacks were sometimes precipitated by certain movements of the neck. A special X-ray test revealed the cause to be a narrowing of one of the main arteries in the neck supplying blood to the brain. Delicate vascular surgery was considered, but was finally ruled out by the presence of generalized arterial degeneration, though the broad feeling of our group was that in 10 years time, with greater experience and technical prowess, our surgeons might well operate on just such a case, despite her advanced age.

The second patient was an 81-year old ex-wharf labourer who had spent many of his early years working in cotton mills and asbestos factories. His complaint was breathlessness, and he had a long series of elaborate tests to show that he suffered from a fibrosing condition of the lungs which prevented oxygen from getting into his blood stream properly. The extensive debate about this patient was whether he should be put on cortisone or not, as cortisone can sometimes help to delay the laying down of fibrous tissue. My feeling was that this man's lung disease had been progressing over at least 40 years, and that cortisone was not likely to reverse the ravages of the decades. Moreover, long-term use of cortisone can have serious side-effects, particularly in old people. Though this view held the day, it was opposed with great vigour and conviction by some of my very able younger colleagues.

These two cases exemplify many of the dilemmas of modern medical practice: the relentless trend towards greater complexity in diagnosis and treatment; the ultra-specialization of medicine; the conflict between a desire to exercise a technological skill and a desire not to meddle uselessly against natural senescence; the increasing importance of geriatrics; the escalating costs of advanced health care; the dangers of depersonalization inherent in a hospital system. They highlight the need for extensive re-thinking of patterns of medical practice. In this chapter, we must look at how research knowledge has changed, is changing, and will continue to change the face of health care delivery systems. We must look first at preventive medicine and then at the progressively more difficult areas of curative and supportive medicine.

## Prevention is better than cure

The most successful type of medical research is that resulting in the development of effective preventive measures. The cardinal examples come from the fields of infectious disease (vaccination, hygienic improvements) or nutrition (elimination of vitamin deficiencies and optimization of growth and development), but scores of less dramatic prophylactic steps have been uncovered by research. Examples such as the relationship between smoking and lung cancer; between excess sugar or insufficient fluoride and dental caries; or between obesity and many diseases spring readily to mind. An area which is closely related to outright prevention is that of early diagnosis of disease, while the patient is still free of, or unaware of, symptoms. School medical services to detect cardiac murmurs, defects in vision or hearing, and many other correctable abnormalities, play a big role in modern health care delivery, and one which is certain to be expanded as research gives greater insight into disease causation and progression. This much is non-controversial, and one can confidently expect that as major developments in medical science generate worthwhile prophylactic measures, the state will, with lag-times reflecting the nature of the particular society, set up a machinery to confer that benefit on its citizens. What is more controversial is the role that multiphasic screening of adults should play in a modern health care system.

## Multiphasic screening and health check-ups

Attitudes towards routine health checks must depend first on the nature of the check to be performed. Few could quarrel, for example, with the common sense approach taken by most life insurance companies. This involves a simple history and physical examination, including testing for high blood pressure and obvious diabetes. While these examinations, and those of prospective employers, are usually geared to the interests of the organization concerned, rather than to the welfare of the person being screened, they can nevertheless help community health by alerting people to their problems. Furthermore, an occasional chat with a medical practitioner can help to transfer useful information about minor health problems. The real problem arises when the proposed check-up involves elaborate X-rays and blood tests, and various forms of internal examination designed to detect early cancer. Many so called 'executive check ups' cost upwards of $300 to perform and involve as much as a full day of the patient's time. Some firms demand this kind of test each six months, and a cost-benefit analysis of the process seems in order.

The trouble is that we still know little of the pre-clinical stages of most serious human illnesses. It is established that the sufferer from human coronary artery disease often has a higher blood cholesterol level than a non-coronary person of the same age and sex. It is likely, but not proven beyond doubt, that a reduction in the amount of animal fats in the diet can reduce blood cholesterol and perhaps slow down the progress of coronary disease. However, many patients with moderately elevated blood cholesterol levels never develop coronary disease. How much trouble should one take to persuade all men over 35 to have blood cholesterol check-ups? How hard should one plead with those that have elevated levels but are quite healthy to change their life style? How much human distress and neurotic pre-occupation with health will one produce in the meantime? The answers are far from clear in the present state of medical knowledge. The same theme could be developed for cancer check-ups. New and more elaborate cancer screening tests are being developed. We ourselves are working on a sensitive radio-isotope method which, hopefully, could develop into an early warning test for cancer of the intestine and certain other cancers. Yet, in many ways, such tests, at least in their early stages, pose more problems than they solve. Suppose a whole population were screened, and the tests on all positive persons were repeated to exclude an error in labelling or technique. Suppose even that the technique were so good as to yield no 'false positives' – something which applies to very few tests indeed in biomedical science. We would be left with a group of people with tiny cancers, possibly curable by surgery. The trouble is, we would not know where the cancer was. We might X-ray every part of the body; we might repeat every conceivable test at three-monthly intervals. When would the time come that we perform our first exploratory operation? How many people will we drive to the brink of suicide in the process. In practical terms, the 'false negatives' in a screening programme can be equally troublesome; consider the patient with a negative cancer test who nevertheless manifests the disease some months later.

These simple examples lead to two obvious conclusions about multiphasic screening or indeed all other forms of health screening of large population groups. First, one must be exceedingly cautious about screening programmes arising from dubious motives. Enormous amounts of money can be made in this area, and exploitation of basic human fears is a real possibility. Secondly, serious screening procedures should initially be regarded as experiments, and the endeavour should be linked to a substantial research base. Indeed, surveys of whole human populations for various biometric parameters have immense potential value for future medical research. We will *never* know the real predictive value of a high blood cholesterol until large numbers of people from diverse socioeconomic, ethnic and geographical backgrounds, *without* evidence of coronary artery disease, have their blood cholesterol tested *and* have regular health examinations for the next 10 to 20 years. The build-up of this kind of information, though aided greatly by computers, is still agonizingly difficult, slow and expensive. It is all the more important that such screening as is done in the world today be part of a well-designed master plan. It is difficult to escape the conclusion that most of the elaborate health screening programmes which exist today fail to meet these criteria. The worst of them are little more than 'gimmicks', and unfortunately these can easily detract from the more serious epidemiological projects that may be going on in the same city.

We are in a half-way house situation about health screening at the present time. We do not yet have the system designed that can optimize use of the information gathered. We do have some tests of sufficient promise to warrant continued effort, thought and debate around the subject. It may well be that quite an elaborate series of automated tests of health will eventually seem just as routine as the yearly visit to the dentist. However, in my view this time will not arrive before the end of the century.

## Delivery of curative and supportive medicine

The much bigger problem area is that of the delivery of health care to people when illness actually strikes them. Here much of the new complexity arises directly from medical research. New, elaborate and expensive diagnostic techniques have emerged; new and ultraspecialized treatment methods (such as coronary care units or kidney transplants) have been developed and are being clamoured for by more and more communities. At the same time, the 'bread and butter' medicine – the boils, the sore throats, the aching backs, the delivery of babies – must still be dispensed in an efficient manner. Furthermore, both the proportion and the absolute number of people living to an advanced age are increasing, and thus geriatric problems are placing bigger demands on the system. Additional factors in the escalating costs of health care are the apparent rise in psychological and social medical problems; the need for better rehabilitation facilities; and the rises in salaries of nursing, paramedical and medical workers. With all of these factors, delivery of optimal medical services has become a problem of enormous dimensions.

The essence of the problem is how to get the right level and kind of professional skill to the particular patient in the most efficient manner. Almost any doctor or nurse can give an injection or take out stitches. It takes a little more, but only a little more, expertise to lance a boil or remove a simple foreign body from the eye. To operate safely on an inflamed appendix requires distinctly more experience again, but this procedure in its turn cannot compare with a complex thoracic or neurosurgical operation. It is not efficient for the top, experienced surgeon to be involved in simple appendectomies, nor for the fourth year surgical registrar, good at appendectomies, to spend time taking routine blood samples. Apart from the issue of level of skill, there is the even more important one of *kind* of skill. The fourth year surgical registrar will be efficient at solving a very different set of problems from those facing the fourth year trainee psychiatrist. How, then, do we achieve a balanced, pyramidal approach employing the time-honoured management principle that decisions should be taken at the lowest safe level?

The matter is made more complex by the fact that people are people, and not machines with broken parts. On the one hand, the patient may feel that he can afford to take his problem to a 'good man', and may be reluctant to accept the fact that a paramedical worker may be well qualified to solve it. On the other hand, doctors are human, too, anxious to test their skills to the limit, to 'hang on' to interesting cases, and at times prone to overestimate their ability or even more frequently to underestimate the advantages of an ultraspecialized opinion (see Chapter 9 for some examples).

## The role of the general practitioner

Different countries have developed differing systems of health care delivery and it is clear that no community has evolved a method which is so superior as to completely satisfy both the patients and the doctors. I believe that the most satisfactory systems are those rooted in a community, and set up specifically to serve its needs, rather than those allowed to evolve largely around the medical profession itself. A first goal towards which one might strive is to ensure that the doctor of first contact, usually the general practitioner or his equivalent, lives a significant part of his professional life attached to a hospital or clinic. This simple step is the biggest single key to the maintenance of adequate personal professional standards. No one wishes to look incompetent in front of his peers. A vibrant relationship between the community hospital and local general practitioners would also further intelligent use of paramedical personnel, and would facilitate both specialist referrals and patient after-care. Geographical considerations can play a big role. The simple expedient of having most of the general practitioners' consulting rooms attached to the community clinic could alone ensure the desired contact, but would clearly be less practical for widely-dispersed suburban or rural communities. A competing concept to the community health centre is the private group practice. Here, several general practitioners, joined perhaps by a paediatrician, a surgeon and an obstetrician, group together to provide a more satisfactory service than that given by a solo practitioner. Unless the group gets very large, however, in which case it really comes to resemble the community clinic, it is inevitable that the specialist members of the group will be caught up in routine duties; in time the edge might go off their specialty skills. The community hospital could usually be large enough to draw on full-time physicians, surgeons and other specialists for both inpatient and consultative care.

It is frequently said that the day of the general practitioner has passed; that there is no longer a need for him; and that patients will increasingly make their way to specialists of their own accord. I disagree with this view, because in many instances the patient is a very poor judge of what ails him. I do believe, however, that the role of the general practitioner must change progressively, so much so that general practice could become a new specialty in its own right. There will be a bigger commitment to social medicine, to community health education, to problems of disease in a total human setting. Due weight will be given to elements such as psychological factors, family, occupation and environment. The new style GP will be strong in human biology, basic psychiatry, geriatrics and, hopefully, on old-fashioned virtues such as charity and common sense. He will increasingly see himself *not* as the slick occasional surgeon or the handy anaesthetist, but as the health advisor with a deep community commitment, a broad and balanced view of medicine, and an efficient liaison system with his specialists. Within this framework, there is unlimited scope for research and imaginative development. A general practitioner with a post-graduate interest in social medicine could lead a rich and enormously useful life, while never lifting a scalpel nor needing to remember the correct dose of the latest blood pressure pill. His human involvement with the families in his district, and his instinct to look beyond the merely mechanistic aspects of organic disease will be the factors that prevent him from becoming merely a referral clerk.

Maybe a good guide to the limits of the general practitioner's executive actions could be provided by what I call the 'doctor's wife' rule. Few doctors would, for preference, see a solo general practitioner remove their wife's appendix or uterus, or deliver her baby, or assume total management of her diabetes or hypertension. These and most other major medical procedures are the responsibility of specialists. If the solo general practitioner is not acceptable, today, for the doctor's wife, he will not be acceptable, tomorrow, for the increasingly educated general citizen. Most doctors that I know, however, do have their own personal general practitioners. What do they use them for? To help in a great diversity of common health problems – childhood infections; chronic illnesses which, despite the specialist's diagnosis and management plan, still need day to day attention; routine health services and check-ups; all manner of minor reassurances; advice as to the quality of available specialists; support in post-operative management and rehabilitation; planning of geriatric care. Most doctors, in fact, admire and value a *good* general practitioner who accepts the challenge of his own *metier* and does not try to do bits of the work of ten specialists. Looked at singly, the tasks listed above may sound trivial, but added together they require real ability and can give real satisfaction.

## Ancillary personnel

The technological revolution in medicine, fed by research, has proven very expensive, and the doctor's personal remuneration is, in many communities, a large factor in the overall cost structure. Society will demand that the doctor husbands his time effectively. It is clear that many aspects of private practice act against efficient utilization of paramedical workers, and especially of nurses, social workers and therapists. These workers have, in general, been trained in and through a hospital system and are only beginning to exercise their proper role in ambulatory and domiciliary medical care. In many countries, there are fiscal barriers to the efficient use of such people, as one can recoup doctor's fees, but not paramedical fees, through insurance schemes. It seems likely that in countries where a fee for service system is the basis for medical remuneration, the pressures for doctors to continue to give services that might more properly be given by a paramedical worker will remain considerable. Much thought should be given to ways of reducing overall health costs and improving standards of care by wider deployment of these ancillary services.

## The larger hospital

The community hospital, with adequate specialist staff, should be able to cope with many of the problems funnelled to it by the doctor of first contact. These include obstetric care, minor to moderate surgery, and management of the common internal diseases. A big advantage of the smaller community hospital is that it is not as impersonal and frightening as the large hospital with its many ultra-specialized units. The smaller place can more readily maintain a happy, comforting atmosphere, *esprit de corps* amongst the staff, and a sense of community involvement. However, inevitably patients will be identified that need more specialized and elaborate care. Major surgery, management of rare diseases, serious problems arising in subspecialty fields such as dermatology, neurology, ophthalmology and so forth, all require referral from the community hospital to a central, more 'high-powered' specialized clinic, which drain substantially larger population areas.

Much controversy exists about the best organization for these major hospitals. Some favour very large hospitals, with 1000 to 2000 beds, where every specialty is duly represented. Others argue for moderate sized hospitals with 500–800 beds, and some rationalization such that one hospital chooses to develop cardiac surgery, another neurosurgery, another kidney transplants, and so forth. A third view, not currently popular, is that each hospital in this central group be very highly specialized, one centre dealing only with accidents; the next only with ear, nose and throat; the next only with chest problems. All manner of compromises between these three versions exist in different countries.

There is, however, general agreement about some of the chief difficulties faced in this area of high-powered medical care. The depersonalizing aspects, seen most clearly in the very large centres, are only too obvious. Correct application of elaborate, science-based medical procedures will take the patient from the comforting care of his general practitioner. He must, in fact, enter the medical mill. He has to work his way through a maze of uncomfortable or even painful diagnostic tests. He encounters the inevitable coterie of residents, registrars and students, whose unfamiliar presence may make him think he is particularly ill. All too frequently, the head of the clinic, to whom the patient has really been referred, is an extremely hard-working, stressed individual, possibly a leader in his field, with international responsibilities. He may not always take the time for the friendly chit-chat which can so greatly smooth the patient's path. The more advanced and research-oriented the unit, the greater the need to assess the patient in detailed quantitative terms and to regard him as a case that will make part of a publishable series. The more renowned the group, the more young doctors are attracted to it, and the more its functioning becomes that of a team. The relationship can easily change from that of individual patient and individual guide, philosopher and friend to that of interesting case and prestigious group. These factors will tax both the common sense of the patient and the tact of the specialists.

Another interesting feature of the medical mill is its all or none quality. You cannot be 'half-in' a teaching hospital. When you go in, the mill grinds on inexorably. For serious or trivial case alike, the history is taken by student, resident, registrar and honorary in relentless progression; the rigmarole of pulse charts, blood tests, X-rays, urine collection must unfold with preordained precision. I mentioned a moment ago the concept of common sense. This quality is *not* a hall-mark of the teaching hospital viewed as a collective whole. As in any large organization, there are inevitably people who find it easier to follow routines (ordering the unnecessary blood test, giving the unwanted sleeping pill) than to use common sense. Thus every trip to a major hospital becomes a 'performance', and the decision to send a patient there one by no means to be taken lightly.

## Virtues in ultra-specialization

What I have said so far sounds negative, but indeed is intended only as a cautionary tale told by a devil's advocate. I mention these dangers of depersonalization only because I am convinced they can be overcome by greater awareness. As a research man, I am, of course, passionately committed to the goal of better health through science and technology, and thus to the vision of the ultra-specialist as the agent who brings research dreams to life. I recall a remark which I heard Sir Ernst Chain attribute to Louis Pasteur, but which I have not been able to trace to its original source. Pasteur is said to have advised his disciples to stick to a single line of research for a long period of years, for only in this way would they develop an 'instinct for truth'. How aptly that phrase describes much of the functioning of the expert! If you treat diabetics all day, every day, you come to *know* which patient needs insulin and which does not. If you operate on the abdomen 10 times per week, you *know* where the common bile duct runs and how not to cut it accidentally! Each of us, through specialization, develops his own 'instinct for truth', his own complement of confident reflex responses. I am sure it will not surprise anyone to hear that though the gifted generalist is still respected and even envied, the vast bulk of documented advances in medicine and science is attributable to full-time careerist, highly-focussed specialists with years of training and experience in their chosen field. Time and again, mortality and morbidity statistics prove that life-threatening diseases are best handled by such groups. Time and again, the complex nature and rapid change of modern medical problems dictate the need for a trained 'in-group', that speaks the jargon, taps the grapevine, culls efficiently the unwieldly literature, brings the 'good oil' to the individual patient. So ultra-specialization is here to stay, and we must now learn to reap maximum benefits from its advantages, while learning to adapt to its disadvantages and limitations.

Another difficulty in ultra-specialization relates to teaching of medical students. By tradition, the clinical teaching is done *not* in community hospitals but in the large, research-oriented centres. This can give students an atypical, unbalanced view of disease patterns. The more specialized that such hospitals become, the graver the problem. Ways will have to be worked out for involving the peripheral community hospitals more in the teaching process, perhaps by some form of affiliation with the larger centres.

## The maintenance of individual dignity in the medical mill

We must briefly return to the dilemma of the two patients described at the beginning of this chapter. It is still an agonizingly difficult task to decide when the medical mill should grind on and when the wise counsellor should rise up and say: 'desist'. In this situation, there are no easy answers. A major part of the burden falls on the biocrat himself. However ultrascientific his clinical duties may be, he must constantly and consciously strive to protect his patient's dignity and to preserve an aura of human warmth, and personal concern. It is clear that the human aspects of medical care need constant and heavy stressing in our curricula. The patient, too, must play his part in making the new kind of doctor-patient relationship a realistic one in this more complex age. I suspect that the days when patients looked on doctors as little tin gods have already gone forever. Nevertheless, I am still frequently amused at the way many individuals decry the medical profession as a whole, while stoutly extolling the virtues of *their particular doctor*. The patient must become used to the idea of his doctor as the head of a team, as an individual whose effectiveness is dependent on a fluctuating nexus of connections with both colleagues and institutions. The patient must be educated to accept some degree of impersonal processing by the medical mill as a reasonable price for more accurate diagnosis and more informed care.

## The cost of health care delivery and medical research

Escalating health costs are worrying every developed nation. They amount to 5 to 8 per cent of the gross national product, and are rising at a faster rate than GNP. To an extent, medical research fans this rate of increase by providing increasingly elaborate tests and treatments. However, that statement tells only part of the story – the pessimistic part. In a very real sense, the hope of curbing escalating health costs rests in medical research.

One can divide medical procedures, as previously indicated, into three types: preventive, curative and supportive. Preventive measures are the best fruits of medical research on all counts: they confer the greatest human benefits and, in general, are rather cheap. Curative medicine, where swift and straightforward medical or surgical intervention solves particular health problems in a definitive way as they come up, is the next best thing to prophylaxis. It may involve considerable expense, but this is of limited duration and the patient can quickly return to normal life and productivity. By far the most expensive results of medical research are what one might term the *partially* successful advances. Here, elaborate procedures are undertaken which have been found to be of help in chronic problems, but which ameliorate rather than cure. The patient remains under medical scrutiny for long periods, some of them spent in hospital. His productivity may remain diminished. He may require various drugs for a lifetime. All the factors add to the total health bill.

It remains the aim of medical research to shift emphasis continually from support to cure to prevention. As recently as the 19th century, medicine could contribute little but symptomatic support. Cure was left to nature and prevention was almost unknown. The greater the degree of fundamental understanding of causative mechanism of disease, the more likely does intelligent control of disease become. Such knowledge rarely arrives in a blinding flash; there may be long periods of partial insight when the best that can be offered is valuable but far from ideal help. Before we had a polio vaccine, long-term respirators were necessary; before streptomycin, tuberculosis sanatoria fulfilled a need; before the dangers of maternal rubella or thalidomide intake were recognized, the handicapped children did need permanent support. Should we forget the economic lessons learnt from these triumphs? Care of the stroke and cancer patient, maintenance of kidney transplant recipients, supportive nursing of chronic nervous system disease all take heavy toll of our health care facilities today. Many of these available expensive treatment measures are the direct results of medical research. Should we castigate the research man for making things so expensive? Or should we rather urge him to press on at full speed, so that the partial measures now available become superseded in their turn?

In this era of instant global communications, social attitudes spread rapidly and can become very stereotyped. When I was a fresh graduate in the middle 1950's, all my brighter colleagues looked unhesitatingly to medical research as the idealist's solution to the major health problems. Today, the pendulum has swung too far the other way. The idealistic young men are all saying: 'we know enough, but must apply it to the less privileged amongst us'. They are eschewing research in favour of more direct community involvement. I would be the last to begrudge adequate care to poor people, but I do contest the claim that research has done its job. We remain woefully ignorant of the causes of many diseases. We have had a pretty good century or so in scientific medicine, but we are really just beginning. To doubt the long-term potential of research at this point is surely to ignore history. Indeed, the very changes in patterns of health care delivery that today's idealists are urging can only come about through research. We need scientific information that can convince politicians of the need for change, and experimental schemes than can serve as models for more definitive restructuring. The problem of organization of medical services is a scientific one just as much as it is a social one. Let our best young doctors remain people with a deep commitment, but let them also remember that their goals will be achieved only through the rigorous application of scientific principles, at all levels of medical problem-solving.

*Further reading*

Dubos R., *Man, Medicine and Environment*. Praeger, New York (1968).

Dubos R., *Mirage of Health. Utopias, Progress and Biological Change*. Harper Brothers, New York (1959).

Knowles J. H., ed., *Hospitals, Doctors and the Public Interest*. Harvard University Press, Cambridge, Mass. (1965).

# 13

# Science and the human condition

'*To deride the hope of progress is the ultimate fatuity, the last word in poverty of spirit and meanness of mind*'. Sir Peter Medawar, 1969.

Two themes dominate the vast quantity of material that has been written about the effects of science and technology on mankind. The first we may term the Huxley-Orwell death of the human spirit theme. The second has so many verbally prolific exponents that an accurate eponymic description would fill a chapter by itself, so let us simply term it the ecodisaster theme. Writers of the former school assure us that science and technology have solved or will solve so many problems that the zest and point will go out of life. The implication is that when there is no need for hard work, no struggles for food, sex, good health or material prosperity; when scientific processes permeate all aspects of existence, the human spirit as we have known it throughout history will die. The ecodisaster theme tells us that not the human spirit but human survival is threatened. It claims that science has created so many problems that, through over-population, pollution and exhaustion of earth crust resources, society will founder, finally to disappear amidst some explosive cataclysm.

It is not part of my purpose to add to this bulky and, in the main, gloomy literature. However, as medical research is clearly only a part of the wider scientific scene, some reference to the outstanding socio-scientific issues should be made.

I do not know of a single scientist who disputes that population control is the world's number one problem. 1974 has been declared the United Nations Population Year, and the Third World Conference on Population, shortly to be held, will address itself to all aspects of the problem. There is, however, great debate about ways of tackling it and prospects for progress. Some place emphasis on the need for medical research to provide still better, simpler methods of birth control than those currently available. Others are convinced that present methods are nearly adequate, but would like to see a 'back-up' technique whereby a pill could be taken or a tampon inserted which could produce a very early abortion, for example 2 or 3 days after the first missed menstrual period. This seems very close if the prostaglandins live up to their early promise. A very few scientists adopt the extreme position that the choice of how many children a person may have should be taken out of the hands of the individual and assumed by the state. They are so struck by the certainty of impending calamity as to dream of viruses or chemicals added to the water supply that lower median human fertility. There appears to be no room for argument about the urgent need for mass community education about the population problem, and in that respect the more extreme prophets of doom could be said to be exerting a helpful influence. At least they stimulate extra thought and discussion. The great pity is that the type of individual likely to go to a lecture by Paul Ehrlich or to read a report from the Club of Rome is not the one needing to be convinced of the gravity of the problem. Nevertheless, it is heartening to see that the message of the urgency of population control is spreading rather rapidly.

In most discussions on this topic, prime emphasis is given to Asia or South America. However, population growth restraint is equally important in the affluent nations, as the per capita consumption and pollution is so much greater in such countries. A recent report published by the U.S. National Population Commission, a 24-member body headed by Mr. John D. Rockefeller, castigated governmental policies biased in favour of procreation. The report suggests that the present U.S. birth rate, now averaging 2.5 children for each woman, should be reduced to 2.11 children. Even though such a reduction could bring population growth to a halt, the present age-constitution in the U.S.A. is such that it would take 70 years to reach the plateau. The report emphasizes the commission's belief that the goal can be achieved without coercion, and without detriment to the economy. Indeed, it is clear that several European countries have achieved zero population growth already.

While continued research on better methods of birth control is necessary, it may be even more useful to study the moral, social and cultural imperatives that underlie population growth patterns. It is pleasing to note that the World Health Organization, in the policy governing its expanded programme of research on human reproduction, fully recognizes the importance of cultural factors, and the need to provide a wide variety of birth control measures to fit in with the diverse demands of race, religion, educational status and national heritage. There is real need for interdisciplinary research here, as the medical biological side is clearly only one part (and probably not the most important part) of a very complex problem. If such social science research uncovers the reasons for people having large families, a birth control campaign aimed at such a population could be mounted in much more intelligent and incisive fashion. Some aspects of the problem are so self-evident as not to require research. For example, for a poor person leading a restricted, boring life, the affection of and for his or her children may represent virtually the only genuine, lasting joy in that life. Persuasion to restrict family size for the possible future good of the race as a whole is clearly most difficult in such a case. Like so many issues, the one of birth control cannot be viewed in isolation.

The earth crust resources problem focuses chiefly on food, power and minerals. Experts differ on the acuteness of the food problem, though it is generally felt that the green revolution, due to the development of superior genetic strains of various crops, has bought mankind a short respite from large-scale famine. What proportion of the world's arable land is already under optimal cultivation? This also cannot be answered, because it is too much tied up with the question of irrigation, which in its turn centres on availability and cost of power. A further unknown is the long-range potential of the sea for food production, though this is clearly also not infinite. With respect to power, there seems to be more general consensus amongst the relevant scholars. Fossil fuels such as oil, natural gas and coal will run out within 50–100 years. Conventional nuclear power dependent on uranium would last much longer, but may not be necessary. First, fast breeder reactors that generate more fissionable material than they use are nearing practicability. Secondly, the prospects of harnessing nuclear fusion, as in the hydrogen bomb, for energy production seem promising. Two other exciting long-range possibilities for power are solar energy, where the chief problems seem to relate to materials technology with respect to the proposed radiation-capturing surfaces, and the fuel cell. Once some or all of these non-polluting, non-exhaustible energy sources become economic realities, the impact on food production, using desalination and other irrigation approaches, will be considerable. As regards minerals, there seems little agreement on how close to exhaustion we may be. The uncertainty relates to the vast areas not yet geologically surveyed, and to the economics of tapping deposits with low-grade mineralization. Also plastics technology is advancing rapidly and producing substitute materials. Many scientists feel that fossil fuels are far too valuable to burn, and should soon be used primarily as raw materials for plastics. Also, it is evident that recycling of materials in consumer durables, particularly automobiles, should become a universal practice.

An important thought to inject is that man is not the only species with a right to inhabit the planet. As the percentage of the earth's surface needed to feed him, or indeed the percentage of the incident solar radiation harnessed and diverted to his particular requirements, increase progressively, so the amounts available for the myriad of other plant or animal life forms diminish. The prolific diversity of nature, both living and non-living, is self-evidently a prime factor lending value and meaning to human life. Too great an encroachment by man on what little wilderness remains cannot fail to be a self-defeating exercise. This simply brings us back to the overriding importance of global population control.

For most of this century, both capitalist and socialist nations have been mesmerized by the concept of economic growth. In political circles, growth in gross national product has been practically equated with growth in human happiness. The stage has now been reached where it is clear that the problems posed by further growth, at least on a global scale, cancel out the benefits achieved by that growth. A most persuasive analysis of this subject has been made by a group of scientists at the Massachusetts Institute of Technology, headed by D. H. Meadows and their book *Limits to Growth* (see reference list) should be obligatory reading for all educated people. This book points out that, sooner or later, all exponentially growing systems must reach a natural limit. Limits to human growth are provided by the essentially finite nature of every resource on spaceship earth. The authors argue for a basic change of values and goals at individual, national and world levels. Attempts should be made by rational planning of global dimensions to reach a society in an enduring state of economic and ecological equilibrium. It is admitted that such a turning away from consumption-oriented materialism would require a revolution of Copernican dimensions. The hope is expressed that a society released from struggling with growth-caused problems such as pollution and mass starvation would have more energy and ingenuity available to promote progress in activities that do *not* require irreplaceable resources. Education, art, music, religion, basic scientific research, athletics and all forms of social interaction could flourish. The end result could be growth in that elusive entity, quality of life.

The question of the environment and curbing of pollution also has a vital cost element. Widespread use of science and technology has brought us the pollution problem, and there is no doubt that most of the scientific know-how for the control of this pollution already exists. The question is how much society is prepared to pay for a clean environment. For example, electric cars may cost more and be less convenient. Goods manufactured in non-polluting factories may be substantially more expensive than the identical product made by an old-fashioned factory with a conventional smoke-stack. The scientist, perhaps feeling guilty about his role in the environment crisis, stands poised to help, but the massive onslaught on the problem which is required will only begin when social attitudes change and *demand* clear air, clean water and a beautiful countryside. In the short term, it is unlikely that the voices of the conservation-minded minority will have too much practical impact. What is therefore needed is firm and courageous government legislation, particularly with respect to new industrial plants.

Will science ever be able to do anything about war and human aggression? We referred briefly to mind control in Chapter 10 and emphasized how far we still are from a profound understanding of the human nervous system. Nevertheless, the partial insights which we do possess foreshadow the probability of quite terrifying powers. For example, in the experimental rat, a brain area has been identified as the 'pleasure centre'. One can introduce a thin wire into the middle of this centre through the skull and can arrange for the rat itself to decide to stimulate this centre by pressing a lever. This sends an electric current rushing to the pleasure centre. Numerous trials showed that rats would press such a lever in preference to one that yielded them food. In fact, given the chance, the rats would just keep on pressing the pleasure lever until they dropped from exhaustion. Who would care to contemplate the nature of a human society where an equivalent procedure were both possible and practiced? Man already has a variety of drugs which can produce euphoria, and scientific knowledge gained about the human brain will continue to add possibilities of this nature. In the same vein, it could well produce non-toxic chemicals that ablate aggression. However, what we know about the presently-available chemical substitutes for real human experiences, and the ghastly social and medical problems that their widespread use have posed, must surely make us hope that this is a path which mankind chooses not to explore too extensively. The threat is real and the long-term outcome not easy to predict.

Science has contributed to the war problem in an entirely different way. In many branches of science, progress now depends on very effective international information and collaboration networks. The scientific community has readily adapted itself to the concept of one world. The prospect of an effective world government addressing itself to prevention of wars and preservation of spaceship earth strikes most people as hopelessly utopian. Yet, is it not possible that what has already been achieved on a scientific plane might one day be feasible on a political one? The UN General Assembly is a fiasco, yet WHO, UNESCO and FAO really do function in a remarkably effective way within the constraints of their limited budgets. The international research organizations such as

CERN or IARC have encountered no serious difficulties, and have allowed new and more ambitious patterns of research to emerge. In fact, the national differences in background, outlook and temperament that, historically, have been causes of prejudice and war are now clearly recognized as sources of both strength and pleasure within the international scientific community. As scientific ways of thinking seep further into politics, it may not be entirely fatuous to hope that international initiatives positively helpful to man's survival, and embodying the above principles, come forward in increasing numbers. The prevention of wars seems to me much more plausible than it did 20 years ago.

There is no question that the ecodisaster prophets and the 'death of the human spirit' school both base their predictions on problems that are real, massive and urgent. To pretend otherwise, to adopt a bland *insouciance* towards the frightening by-products of the scientific age, would be totally irresponsible. Yet I wonder whether the pervasive pessimism about man's future is warranted. Are there not two sides to the question of science and the human spirit? What about the lightening of crushing work burdens? What about universal education? What about the liberating influence of the realization of man's extraordinary power? What about the sheer beauty revealed as science discovers nature's pattern and order? We have really not had very long to give science a try as a provider of guide-lines to a way of life. Our social interrelationships have been developing over several thousand years, but science has been a major factor in human life for, at most, two centuries. Why not take the view that man's history is just beginning rather than nearly ending? Science has released many minds from ignorance, prejudice and superstition, revealing an incredible reservoir of inventiveness and creativity. This surely gives us at least a fighting chance to make a better world!

It is curious how unpopular – almost disreputable – it has become to be an optimist about the course of history, and the role of science in particular. Yet, a dispassionate assessment surely reveals many science-based activities that contain at least some seeds of hope. The technical experts keep patiently hammering away at the Strategic Arms Limitation Talks. New agreements have recently been signed about international cooperation in space exploration and cancer research. The first Stockholm Conference on the Human Environment produced a modest but significant improvement in the outlook for eventual global pollution control. The creation by the Nobel Foundation of an International Federation of Institutes for Advanced Study is another timely event. This Federation plans to harness the resources of thirty or so of the world's leading research institutes, covering a wide variety of disciplines, towards a frontal attack on the outstanding human problems of our time. In other words, people are not *behaving* as though there were no hope; rather they appear to believe in a positive role for science. Is the pessimism not partly a pose?

Human history is shaped by both thought and action. Human thought evolves slowly but with a relentlessness that seems to brook no retreat. I do not think that man either can or wishes to retreat from science and to re-enter Arcadia. Human action is not always subjugated to thought, and can veer erratically in leaps and bounds. The cataclysms of history have resulted from violent actions that contravened the most evolved standards of thought. The most challenging role which science could play in the future is to aid the proper and constructive sequence: thought first, action afterwards. This aspiration itself demands a revolution of a dimension akin to that caused by the major religious movements. The goal is difficult and remote, yet in this age where man has come to wield such immense power, it must be reached. The potential for disaster inherent in capricious, thoughtless action is just too great. Education and the intelligent application of science will contribute critically to the history that we are now all shaping. If this book has enlarged the reader's knowledge of modern science it will have achieved its aim.

*Further reading*

Burnet, F. M. *Dominant Mammal: the biology of human destiny*. Heinemann, Melbourne (1970).

Ehrlich, P. R. and Ehrlich, A. H. *Population, Resources, Environment: issues in human ecology*. W. H. Freeman and Co., San Francisco (1970).

Huxley, A. L. *Brave New World*. Chatto and Windus, London (1952).

Meadows, D. L. et al. eds., *The Limits to Growth*. A Report for the Club of Rome's Project on the Predicament of Mankind. Universe Books, New York (1972).

Monod, J. *Chance and Necessity*. William Collins, London (1972).

Orwell, G. *Nineteen Eighty Four*. Secker and Warburg, London (1949).

Stent, G. S. *The Coming of the Golden Age: a view of the end of progress*. The Natural History Press, New York (1969).

Toulmin, S. *Foresight and Understanding*. An enquiry into the aims of science. Hutchinson, London (1961).

# Index

UNIVERSITY OF BRISTOL
25 NOV 2019
WITHDRAWN
UNIVERSITY OF BRISTOL MEDICINE
75 18469